T0073874

OXFORD HANDBOOK OF

Sleep Medicine

Published and forthcoming Oxford Handbooks

OXFORD HANDBOOK OF
Sleep Medicine

EDITED BY

Guy Leschziner

Consultant Neurologist and Sleep Physician, Guy's and
St Thomas' NHS Hospitals; Professor of Neurology and Sleep
Medicine, Institute of Psychiatry, Psychology and Neuroscience,
King's College London, London, UK

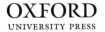

OXFORD
UNIVERSITY PRESS

UNIVERSITY PRESS

Great Clarendon Street, Oxford, OX2 6DP,
United Kingdom

Oxford University Press is a department of the University of Oxford.
It furthers the University's objective of excellence in research, scholarship,
and education by publishing worldwide. Oxford is a registered trade mark of
Oxford University Press in the UK and in certain other countries

First Edition published in 2022

Impression: 1

Published in the United States of America by Oxford University Press
198 Madison Avenue, New York, NY 10016, United States of America

British Library Cataloguing in Publication Data
Data available

Library of Congress Control Number: 2021946453

ISBN 978–0–19–284825–3

DOI: 10.1093/med/9780192848253.001.0001

Printed and bound in China by
C&C Offset Printing Co., Ltd.

Foreword

The field of sleep medicine is very new. When it was born in the early 1970s, sleep disorders were thought to be exquisitely rare, the domain of academic medical centres. The most common disorder, sleep apnoea, did not even receive its name until about 1975. Until the early 1990s, most investigators believed that sleep apnoea did not even occur in women.

A generation later, everybody knows someone with a sleep disorder, and the medical system of most countries has not adapted to deal with a very large number of cases that need diagnosis and treatment. There simply are not enough specialists to deal with the millions of patients with sleep disorders. General practitioners, nurses, and respiratory therapists are playing an increasing important role in managing the patients.

Professor Guy Leschziner and his colleagues have created a magnificent book that takes us into the future of sleep medicine, where the role of the specialist will be, as it should be, to deal with complex and rare sleep disorder cases. The general practitioner is almost always the first caregiver that a patient sees, but patients with sleep disorders will be seen by clinicians or other healthcare professionals in every domain. Doctors should always ask the patient about their sleep, even if this is not their primary complaint. This volume will teach how to interact with the patient, how we elicit important signs and symptoms, and will help the doctor know how to be confident in the diagnosis and management of patients who may not require the services of a specialist, and when to refer for specialist care.

There are over 80 sleep disorders. Most of the common ones are covered in detail in this volume. This book will help both the doctor and the patient. Probably, at least 10% of patients coming into a family doctor's office have a sleep disorder. If a doctor sees 100 patients a week, imagine the 500 patients with sleep disorders that are seen during a year. Imagine how many cases of sleep disorders have been missed, and therefore not treated. This book is an important first step in the meeting this important clinical need.

Meir Kryger, MD, FRCPC
Professor, Yale School of Medicine
Co-Editor, *Principles and Practice of Sleep Medicine*
Author, *Mystery of Sleep*

Contents

Detailed contents

Symbols and abbreviations

➲	cross-reference
🖰	website
~	approximately
AASM	American Academy of Sleep Medicine
AD	Alzheimer's disease
ADHD	attention deficit hyperactivity disorder
AHI	apnoea–hypopnoea index
ASD	autism spectrum disorder
ASWPD	advanced sleep–wake phase disorder
BDI	Beck Depression Inventory
BIISS	behaviourally induced insufficient sleep syndrome
BMI	body mass index
BPAD	bipolar affective disorder
CBT	cognitive behavioural therapy
CBT-I	cognitive behavioural therapy for insomnia
CH	cluster headache
CPAP	continuous positive airway pressure
CRSWD	circadian rhythm sleep–wake disorder
CSA	central sleep apnoea
CSF	cerebrospinal fluid
DAT	dopamine transporter
DLB	dementia with Lewy bodies
DSWPD	delayed sleep–wake phase disorder
EDS	excessive daytime sleepiness
EEG	electroencephalography/ electroencephalogram
EMG	electromyography/ electromyogram
ENT	ear, nose, and throat
EOG	electro-oculography/ electro-oculogram
FOSQ	Functional Outcomes of Sleep Questionnaire
GABA	gamma-aminobutyric acid
$GABA_A$	gamma-aminobutyric acid type A
GAD	generalized anxiety disorder
HbA1c	glycated haemoglobin

HLA	human leucocyte antigen
ICSD-3	International Classification of Sleep Disorders, third edition
IRBD	idiopathic rapid eye movement sleep behaviour disorder
ISWRD	irregular sleep–wake rhythm disorder
KLS	Kleine–Levin syndrome
MAD	mandibular advancement device
MCI	mild cognitive impairment
MDD	major depressive disorder
MRI	magnetic resonance imaging
MSA	multisystem atrophy
MSL	mean sleep latency
MSLT	multiple sleep latency test
Mu2	μ-opioid receptor
MWT	maintenance of wakefulness test
NICE	National Institute for Health and Care Excellence
Non-24	non-24-hour sleep–wake rhythm disorder
NREM	non-rapid eye movement
NT1	narcolepsy type 1
NT2	narcolepsy type 2
OAT	oral appliance therapy
ODI	oxygen desaturation index
OSA	obstructive sleep apnoea
OSAHS	obstructive sleep apnoea/ hypopnoea syndrome
OSLER	Oxford Sleep Resistance Test
PAP	positive airway pressure
PD	Parkinson's disease
PLMD	periodic limb movement disorder
PLMS	periodic limb movements of sleep
PLMW	periodic limb movements of wakefulness
PSG	polysomnography/ polysomnogram
PSM	propriospinal myoclonus
RBD	rapid eye movement sleep behaviour disorder
RDI	respiratory disturbance index
REM	rapid eye movement

RLS	restless legs syndrome
SAQLI	Sleep Apnoea Quality of Life Index
SCN	suprachiasmatic nucleus
SDB	sleep-disordered breathing
SHE	sleep-related hypermotor epilepsy
SNRI	serotonin and norepinephrine (noradrenaline) reuptake inhibitor
SOREMP	sleep-onset rapid eye movement period

SRRMD	sleep-related rhythmic movement disorder
SSRI	selective serotonin reuptake inhibitor
SWS	slow-wave sleep
TSC	tuberous sclerosis complex
UARS	upper airway resistance syndrome
VLPO	ventrolateral preoptic nucleus
vPSG	video polysomnography

Contributors

Romola S. Bucks
Professor, School of Psychological Science, Director, The Raine Study, School of Population and Global Health, University of Western Australia, Perth, Australia

Grainne d'Ancona
Consultant Pharmacist, Sleep Disorders Centre, Guy's and St Thomas' NHS Trust, London, UK

Aditi Desai
President, British Society of Dental Sleep Medicine, London, UK

Panagis Drakatos
Consultant Sleep and Respiratory Physician, Guy's and St Thomas' NHS Trust, London, UK

Sofia Eriksson
Consultant Neurologist, National Hospital for Neurology and Neurosurgery, University College London Hospitals NHS Foundation Trust, London, UK

Michael Farquhar
Consultant in Paediatric Sleep Medicine, Evelina Children's Hospital, Guy's and St Thomas' NHS Trust, London, UK

Valentina Gnoni
Consultant and Sleep Physician, King's College London, London, UK

Paul Gringras
Professor of Paediatric Sleep Medicine, Evelina Children's Hospital, Guy's and St Thomas' NHS Trust, London, UK

Seán E. Higgins
Highly Specialist Sleep Technologist, Guy's and St Thomas' NHS Trust, London, UK

Brian Kent
Consultant Sleep and Respiratory Physician, Guy's and St Thomas' NHS Trust, London, UK

Bhik Kotecha
Consultant ENT Surgeon, Royal National Throat, Nose & Ear Hospital, University College London Hospitals NHS Foundation Trust; Honorary Clinical Professor, Barts and The London School of Medicine and Dentistry, London; Queens Hospital, Romford, UK

Guy Leschziner
Consultant Neurologist and Sleep Physician, Guy's and St Thomas' NHS Trust; Professor of Neurology and Sleep Medicine, Institute of Psychiatry, Psychology and Neuroscience, King's College London, London, UK

Elaine Lyons
Clinical Pharmacist, Sleep Disorders Centre, Guy's and St Thomas' NHS Trust, London, UK

Mary J. Morrell
Professor of Sleep and Respiratory Physiology, National Heart and Lung Institute, Imperial College, London, UK

Rexford Muza
Consultant Sleep and Respiratory Physician, Guy's and St Thomas' NHS Trust, London, UK

Alexander D. Nesbitt
Consultant Neurologist and Sleep Physician, Guy's and St Thomas' NHS Trust, London, UK

David O'Regan
Consultant Psychiatrist and Sleep Physician, Guy's and St Thomas' NHS Trust, Honorary Senior Lecturer, King's College, London, UK

Michelle Olaithe
Clinical Psychologist Honorary Research Fellow, School of Psychological Science, University of Western Australia, Perth, Australia

Ricardo S. Osorio
Associate Professor, Department of Psychiatry, Healthy Brain Aging and Sleep Center (HBASC), New York University Grossman School of Medicine, New York, USA

Laura Pérez-Carbonell
Consultant Neurologist and Sleep Physician, Guy's and St Thomas' NHS Trust, London, UK

Ivana Rosenzweig
Consultant Neuropsychiatrist and Sleep Physician, Guy's and St Thomas' NHS Trust, London, UK

Hugh Selsick
Consultant Psychiatrist, Guy's and St Thomas' NHS Trust, University College London Hospitals, London, UK

Joerg Steier
Professor of Respiratory and Sleep Medicine, Guy's and St Thomas' NHS Foundation Trust and King's College London, UK

Charlie Tyack
Clinical Psychologist, Department of Clinical Psychology and Neuropsychology, Nottingham University Hospitals NHS Trust, Nottingham, UK; Highly Specialist Clinical Psychologist in Paediatric Sleep, Evelina Children's Hospital, Guy's and St Thomas' NHS Trust, London, UK

Adrian J. Williams
Professor of Sleep Medicine, Guy's and St Thomas' NHS Trust, London, UK

Introduction

It is not so long ago that sleep—its functions, its dysfunctions, and its origins—were a mystery. A state of near-death, a metaphysical process, a connection to the spiritual world, perhaps a window into our deep unconscious. Even until very recently, the world of sleep remained a puzzle, not only to scientists but also to clinicians. I do not recall any moment of my medical school education dedicated to sleep and its disorders.

But over the last few years, our understanding of sleep has leapt forward, through advances in scientific techniques and technologies, and the efforts of academic and clinical researchers around the world. We are able to study the sleep and genetics of large cohorts, utilize novel imaging techniques to understand brain function rather than simply structure, and apply a range of research methodologies in the laboratory setting.

In addition to an expanding knowledge of sleep disorders and their management, we are beginning—but only beginning—to comprehend the ramifications of poor or limited sleep on a range of health outcomes: neurological, cardiovascular, immune, psychiatric, respiratory, and pain. And we are also increasingly aware of the bidirectional relationship between a range of medical disorders and sleep, for example, insomnia and depression, or Parkinson's disease and rapid eye movement sleep behaviour disorder. It is becoming apparent that a knowledge of sleep and its disorders is an important tenet of many areas of clinical medicine, and is no longer only of relevance to a few clinicians studying patients in a sleep laboratory.

And, of course, these conditions are not rare curiosities, only to be seen in a specialist clinic. Complaints regarding sleep are one of the commonest issues raised by patients within the primary care setting. Insomnia affects about 30% of the adult population in any 1 year, about 10% on a chronic basis. Obstructive sleep apnoea affects about 1 in 10 adult males, and 1 in 20 adult females, and is increasing in frequency alongside the expansion of our waistlines. Restless legs syndrome affects about 1 in every 20 people. Sleepwalking is so common in childhood as to be considered almost part of the norm, and persists into adulthood in 1–2%. Even narcolepsy, viewed as a rare neurological disorder, has a prevalence of about 1 in 2000; any busy physician is likely to see a few patients with narcolepsy, and most primary practices will be looking after a patient or two with this condition. And in parallel with the medical community's increasing interest in sleep, the general public's awareness of the importance of sleep and of sleep disorders means that more and more people will present to their doctor with these types of problems. Thus, there is a need for an increased understanding of sleep medicine more widely within the medical community, of diagnostic pathways, and treatment strategies.

What this handbook aims to achieve is to arm clinicians with practical basic knowledge of the breadth of sleep disorders they may encounter during their routine clinical practice. How to recognize and diagnose sleep disorders, how to treat them, and when to refer to specialist services. It does not seek to be a definitive reference textbook—there are weightier tomes for that purpose already in existence. We have sought to summarize information that a wide array of clinicians, regardless of background or speciality, will find useful, both with regard to sleep disorders themselves and their interplay with a range of other medical conditions. The book starts with a general introduction to practical sleep medicine, and is divided largely according to type of sleep problems seen—insomnia, hypersomnias (conditions causing excessive sleepiness), and parasomnias (abnormal or unwanted behaviours)—before broadening out into the relevance of these disorders for physical and psychological health and well-being. The following chapters have been written by a wide range of physicians and surgeons, from disparate backgrounds, but all with a keen interest in sleep in all its forms. It exemplifies that sleep is the perfect confluence of physical, psychological, environmental, and behavioural factors that makes the practice of sleep medicine an endlessly fascinating, at times perplexing and frustrating, but ultimately rewarding pursuit.

Guy Leschziner, 2021

The neurobiological basis of sleep

Ivana Rosenzweig

Definition

Sleep is a behavioural state of psychomotor arrest with increased arousal threshold, facilitated by sensory disconnection from the environment. Carskadon and Dement[1] referred to sleep as a recurring, reversible neurobehavioural state of relative perceptual disengagement from, and un-responsiveness to, the environment.

Sleep is commonly accompanied by behavioural quiescence, specific posture, and closed eyes. It encompasses a set of complex, and as of yet not fully understood, interactions in the central nervous system and all other body systems. As humans, we spend up to third of our lives in this universal behavioural state, which has been observed in all animal species.

However, sleep is not merely a passive state in which the brain is quiescent but, rather, a dynamic, highly regulated, and complicated series of brain states that repeat themselves in a characteristic pattern.

The molecular mechanisms that control sleep rhythms are highly conserved phylogenetically. However, the cyclic organization of sleep varies within and between species. The period length of sleep stages appears to increase with brain size across species, and the depth and proportion of the non-rapid eye movement (NREM) stages in each cycle increase with brain maturation within species.

Normal human sleep comprises two major states—rapid eye movement (REM) and NREM sleep, which alternate cyclically during a sleep period:

- NREM sleep includes slowing and increased synchronization of the cortical electroencephalogram (EEG), associated with low muscle tone and minimal cognitive activity. NREM sleep is divided into three stages, according to the degree of synchronization evident on the EEG and other markers:
  - Stage 1 (N1)—drowsiness or light sleep
  - Stage 2 (N2)—intermediate sleep (associated with particular EEG markers such as sleep spindles and K-complexes)
  - Stage 3 (N3)—deep sleep
- REM sleep is characterized by an EEG that is desynchronized, skeletal muscles are atonic (apart from those controlling eye movements), and most dreaming occurs during this stage of sleep
- A nocturnal pattern of sleep commonly includes several reliable characteristics:
  - Sleep begins in NREM N1 and progresses through deeper NREM stages (N2 and N3) before the first episode of REM sleep occurs ~80–100 minutes later
  - After that, NREM sleep and REM sleep cycle with a period of ~90 minutes
  - N3 sleep stages are more concentrated in the early NREM cycles, while REM sleep episodes lengthen across the night
  - Slow-wave sleep (SWS) during N3 predominates in the first third of the night and is linked to the initiation of sleep and the length of time awake

- REM sleep predominates in the last third of the night, and it is linked to the circadian rhythm of body temperature
- Wakefulness in sleep accounts for less than 5% of the night
- NREM sleep is usually 75–80% of sleep
- REM sleep (20–25%) occurs in four to six discrete episodes
- Subsequent sleep following one night of sleep deprivation favours SWS during recovery
- REM sleep rebound occurs on the second or subsequent recovery nights after an episode of sleep loss.

Cortical and, more recently, invasive intracortical patient studies of human sleep have significantly advanced our understanding of sleep electrophysiology. Different sleep oscillations are recognized during NREM and REM recordings, such as slow waves, sleep spindles, gamma and ripple oscillations, and ultraslow neuronal fluctuations. The precise underlying nature and function of these different EEG features is yet to be fully elucidated.

Neuroanatomical and neurotransmitter basis of sleep

The twenty-first century has, with technological advances in molecular biology, genomics, imaging, and neurophysiology, enabled a more complete picture of the cellular mechanisms and subcortical networks that underlie the neurobiology of sleep. However, according to the still influential classical sleep model, the timing and quality of sleep are predominantly determined by intricate coalescence and interplay of *ultradian*, *homeostatic*, and *circadian* factors. In chronobiology, an ultradian rhythm is defined as a recurrent period or cycle repeated throughout a 24-hour day, while circadian rhythms complete one cycle daily.

- The accumulation of an endogenous chemical adenosine in the brain during prolonged wakefulness constitutes the physiological basis of the homeostatic sleep pressure, i.e. the longer one is awake, the stronger the drive to go to sleep. This homeostatic mechanism driving sleep is termed 'Process S' in Borbely's two-process model of sleep propensity
- The second process influencing sleep is that of the circadian rhythm, also referred to as 'Process C'. It is the interaction between these two processes that influences the propensity to fall asleep at any particular time.

These two processes, homeostatic and circadian, are both largely controlled by and regulated in the hypothalamus:

- The *homeostatic 'switch'* for sleep is considered to be located in the brain's ventrolateral preoptic nucleus (VLPO) of the anterior hypothalamus. This area becomes active during sleep and uses the inhibitory neurotransmitter gamma-aminobutyric acid (GABA) and galanin to initiate sleep by inhibiting the arousal regions of the brain:
  - The VLPO is triggered to initiate sleep onset by both circadian input from the anterior hypothalamus and sleep–wake homeostatic information from endogenous chemical signals, such as adenosine, which accumulate in proportion to time spent awake
  - It can inhibit the awake-promoting regions of the brain, distributed throughout the midbrain and brainstem
  - Thus, the VLPO might initiate sleep onset (and the inhibition of REM sleep) through its reciprocal inhibition of cholinergic, noradrenergic, and serotonergic arousal systems in the brainstem. It acts similarly on histaminergic arousal systems of the posterior hypothalamus and cholinergic systems of the basal forebrain
  - According to this sleep model, hypocretin (orexin) neurons in the lateral hypothalamus help to stabilize the 'switch' and when the hypocretin neurons are lost, narcolepsy can result

- The *circadian sleep rhythm* is among several intrinsic body rhythms modulated by the hypothalamus. Circadian rhythmicity is based on an interlocking positive–negative feedback mechanism that controls gene transcription in the suprachiasmatic nucleus (SCN) of the hypothalamus:
  - When light activates distinct cells within the retina (retinal ganglion cells), this causes the SCN to signal the pineal body to stop secreting melatonin
  - The SCN sets the body's 'clock' to ~24.2 hours, with both light exposure and other factors (termed *Zeitgebers*) entraining to the 24-hour cycle
  - SCN cells affect adjacent brain nuclei of the anterior hypothalamus, which in turn entrain other structures that control rhythmic physiological processes, such as sleep, temperature, and endocrine/hormonal output.

Once sleep is initiated, *an ultradian oscillator* in the mesopontine junction of the brain controls the regular alternation of NREM and REM sleep. The executive control of this oscillator involves a reciprocal interaction between REM-on (cholinergic) and REM-off (aminergic) cell groups, whose influence on one another is mediated by interposed excitatory, inhibitory, and autoregulatory circuits. These neuronal circuits are known to involve and other brain chemicals/neurotransmitters such as glutamate, as well as serotonin, noradrenaline, and acetylcholine.

Sleep, synaptic homeostasis, and memory

Prolonged sleep loss is known to lead to cognitive deficits, emotional fragility, and increased neuropsychiatric deficits, as well as increased incidence of neurodegenerative disorders. Sleep deprivation and fragmentation similarly impairs other body organ systems; affects temperature control, metabolism, and immune function; and, when prolonged, may ultimately lead to death.

The core brain function of sleep is still hotly debated. More recently the synaptic homeostasis hypothesis (SHY) by Cirelli and Tononi[2] in 2003 proposed that sleep enables continued brain plasticity during active states of consciousness:

- According to this hypothesis, during wakefulness, synapses undergo net strengthening (potentiation) as a result of adaptive learning during wakefulness and exposure to an ever-changing environment. During sleep, a degree of re-normalization occurs
- This plasticity of the brain is essential for survival, and to enable this metabolically demanding process, sleep provides a crucial state during which our brain is disconnected from the environment, when neural circuits can be reactivated, renormalizing synaptic strength
- This process also enables memory consolidation and the integration of new with old memories, and eliminates the superfluous synapses, as well as restores the homeostasis of energy and cellular supplies, with beneficial effects at both the systems and cellular level.

Another core role for sleep includes the establishment of memories.[3,4] Numerous studies have shown that sleep periods after learning improve memory formation, and sleep likely promotes consolidation and reorganization of memories:

- Both REM and SWS stages support memory processes
- Although the exact mechanisms are unclear, they probably involve replay of stored patterns of brain activity elicited during behaviour and learning that is coupled with synaptic plasticity processes
- The reactivation of memories in the context of hippocampal–neocortical dialogue is thought to occur during deep NREM sleep when it is hypothesized that hippocampal reactivation stimulates redistribution of memory representations to cortical circuitry
- While still controversial, there is evidence in the literature that similarly supports REM sleep's role in consolidation of higher-order abstract memory, and perhaps simultaneously leads to forgetting of episodic memory.

Sleep and the glymphatic system

More recently, the N3 stage of sleep has been linked in animals with a newly discovered macroscopic waste clearance system in the brain that utilizes a unique system of perivascular channels formed by astroglial cells.

This so-called glymphatic system promotes efficient elimination of soluble proteins and metabolites from the central nervous system. It may also help distribution of various compounds in the brain, such as glucose, lipids, and amino acids, and it may aid volumetric transmission of some neurotransmitters.

It is still uncertain whether the glymphatic system in the human brain functions in the same manner to that noted in rodents. Moreover, it is unclear during which sleep stage/s it might function.

Conclusion

The basis of sleep—its initiation, regulation, and behavioural correlates—is neurological, but all available evidence indicates that sleep is restorative for brain function and has a vital role for supporting mood and cognition.

Further reading

Dudai Y, Karni A, Born J. The consolidation and transformation of memory. Neuron. 2015;88(1):20–32.

Hobson JA. Sleep is of the brain, by the brain and for the brain. Nature. 2005;437(7063):1254–6.

Tononi G, Cirelli C. Sleep and the price of plasticity: from synaptic and cellular homeostasis to memory consolidation and integration. Neuron. 2014;81(1):12–34.

References

1. Carskadon M, Dement W. Normal human sleep: An overview. In: Kryger MH, Roth T, Dement WC (Eds) Principles and Practice of Sleep Medicine, 4th ed. Philadelphia, PA: Elsevier Saunders; 2005.
2. Tononi G, Cirelli C. Sleep and synaptic homeostasis: A hypothesis. Brain Research Bulletin. 2003;62(2):143–150.
3. Diekelmann S, Born J. The memory function of sleep. Nature Reviews Neuroscience. 2010;11:114–126.
4. Stickgold R. Sleep-dependent memory consolidation. Nature 2005;437:1272–1278.

Sleep and the glymphatic system

Conclusion

Further reading

References

General approach to sleep disorders

Rexford Muza

Introduction

Taking a good sleep history, evaluating the symptoms appropriately, and developing the necessary diagnostic skills are essential in the management of sleep disorders. As with all other aspects of dealing with medical problems, the usual sequence should be history taking followed by examination, and then coming to a presumptive diagnosis. Further diagnostic formulation is aided by relevant investigations and then a management plan is put in place.

Sleep assessment summary

Sleep history format

- The patient's profile
- Chief complaint/presenting complaint
- History of presenting complaint
- Further sleep history exploration (e.g. sleep schedule, sleep environment, sleep hygiene)
- Past medical history: similar to routine medical work-up
- Psychiatric history: are there current symptoms or a past history of psychosis, depression, anxiety, or personality disorder?
- Family medical history: some sleep disorders have a familial predisposition (e.g. sleep walking, narcolepsy, restless legs syndrome (RLS))
- Social history: occupation—are they a shift or night worker, do they frequently travel across time zones? Do they drive? And if so, what type of licence do they hold and what sort of journeys do they have to do? Do they have any other safety-critical jobs such as flying or operating safety-critical machinery?
- Medications: regular prescription medications as well as over-the-counter and herbal remedies
- Allergies: routine as per good clinical practice
- Systems review: as per usual medical work-up but with emphasis on issues relevant to sleep:
  - Cardiorespiratory symptoms (angina, orthopnoea, paroxysmal nocturnal dyspnoea, etc.)
  - Gastrointestinal symptoms: inquire about heart burn/gastric reflux—symptoms which can disturb sleep
  - Nocturia: can disturb sleep (and is also a feature of obstructive sleep apnoea (OSA))
  - Reduced libido; this can be due to OSA but can also be an important side effect of medications used in the management of sleep disorders
  - Arthritic and other painful conditions will affect sleep.

Physical examination

Emphasis should be directed by the chief complaint:
- Weight/body mass index (BMI)
- Neck collar size (circumference)
- Nasopharynx—examine for nasopharyngeal oedema, turbinate hypertrophy, or a deviated nasal septum
- Oropharynx—the Mallampati score is a useful way of describing oropharyngeal narrowing:
  - Do they have retrognathia?
  - Do they have macroglossia?
  - Do they have enlarged tonsils?
- Cardiac, pulmonary, and neurological examinations (type of examination required is directed by the symptoms).

Taking a sleep history

From a clinical perspective, three main sleep problems are usually encountered:

- Insomnia—inability to get to sleep or stay asleep
- Hypersomnia—prolonged sleep duration, excessive daytime sleepiness (EDS), or difficulty waking up. Examples of causes of EDS include:
  - EDS due to fragmented night sleep as might be the case in OSA and other sleep-disrupting pathologies
  - EDS due to a central hypersomnolence disorder
  - EDS due to a medical disorder
  - EDS due to a psychiatric disorder (e.g. depression)
  - EDS due to drugs
  - Behaviourally induced inadequate night-time sleep
- Parasomnia—abnormal behaviours in or surrounding sleep.

The sleep clinician should be aware of the broader classification as stated in the third edition of the *International Classification of Sleep Disorders* (ICSD-3) which identifies seven major categories of sleep problems:

- Insomnia disorders (→ Chapters 4–6)
- Sleep-related breathing disorders (→ Chapters 7 and 8)
- Central disorders of hypersomnolence (→ Chapters 14 and 15)
- Circadian rhythm sleep–wake disorders (→ Chapter 16)
- Sleep-related movement disorders (→ Chapters 13 and 19)
- Parasomnias (→ Chapters 17–19)
- Other sleep disorders.

History taking aims to delineate symptoms and eventually arrive at a specific sleep disorder. The initial focus should be on taking a thorough history of the presenting complaint from the patient and, ideally, the bed partner or parent/carer. The duration of symptoms and the effects of symptoms on daytime functioning should be explored. It is helpful to attempt to characterize the general category of sleep complaint, before proceeding to a more directed history.

Important aspects of the sleep history include:

- General exploration of sleep patterns:
  - Usual bed time and rise times
  - Estimated sleep latency (time to sleep onset) and duration
  - Number of awakenings
  - Morning symptoms
  - The presence and duration of daytime naps
- Habits:
  - Caffeine consumption—quantity per day, and at what times it is consumed
  - Alcohol use—amount, and how long before bedtime
  - Smoking habits—how much, and how soon before bedtime
  - Use of recreational such as cannabis, cocaine, etc.
- Pre-sleep behaviours:
  - Daytime schedule, work, and stress
  - Exercise
  - Evening routine
  - Food and drink, e.g. chocolate or large meal before bed
  - Light sources in the bedroom from televisions, mobile phones, and tablets

- Nocturnal sleep characteristics:
  - Regular weekday sleep schedule and weekend/holidays sleep pattern
  - Reasons for any awakenings, e.g. going to the toilet, discomfort, pain, and parasomnias
  - Approximate time it takes to return to sleep after any awakening
  - As relevant, explore events around sleep onset and on final awakening.

In the history taking, the clinician should specifically enquire about the following:
- Symptoms before sleep such as:
  - RLS symptoms or other movements at bed times
  - Listlessness, agitation, anxiety, and alertness at bed times
- Symptoms on entry into sleep:
  - Hypnic jerking—common normal physiological experience but can be exaggerated in other patients
  - Levitation
  - Sleep-onset hallucinations
- Symptoms in sleep such as:
  - Snoring
  - Breathing pauses (apnoeas)
  - Gasping
  - Choking
  - Sweating
  - Body movements in sleep—repetitive movements, flailing, grabbing, punching, kicking, jumping, limping
  - Vocalizations—sleep talking, shouting, swearing
  - Dreams and their characteristics
- Daytime symptoms such as:
  - Morning sleep inertia
  - Morning headaches
  - Dry mouth/sore throat
  - EDS
  - Poor concentration levels/brain fog
  - Irritability
  - Tiredness
  - Symptoms suggestive of cataplexy.

Is the predominant picture one of insomnia?

Insomnia can be classified according to the time of night it occurs, although often more than one type can be present:
- Sleep initiation insomnia is most likely to be due to psychophysiological insomnia, with or without psychiatric comorbidities, but may also be caused by:
  - RLS—ask if there are any features such as an urge to move, especially the legs
  - Delayed sleep phase disorder—ask if the patient sleeps a normal duration but wakes up late if allowed to
  - Anxiety or other psychiatric disorders—ask if there is fear of sleep, any specific phobias around sleep, or any past traumas related to the bedroom or sleep

- Sleep maintenance insomnia—is there no problem going off to sleep, but once asleep, do they wake repeatedly? This may simply be a feature of psychophysiological insomnia, but can indicate:
  - OSA or central sleep apnoea (CSA)
  - Periodic limb movement disorder (PLMD)
  - Anxiety/depression
  - Narcolepsy is often associated with fragmented night-time sleep
- Sleep termination insomnia/early morning waking is a biological feature of depression, but may also indicate advanced sleep phase disorder. Clarify if when allowed to sleep without restraint, the patient goes to bed early and wakes early, with a normal sleep duration.

An important clinical feature is whether there is significant daytime sleepiness in the context of insomnia. Patients with organic sleep disorders such as sleep apnoea, PLMD, or circadian rhythm disorders will often be very sleepy, and of course EDS is the cardinal feature of narcolepsy. In contrast, patients with primary insomnia will often complain of extreme daytime tiredness and fatigue, but will often (but not always!) find it very difficult to fall asleep during the day.

Ask about any specific triggers that the patient feels might have precipitated their insomnia.

Are there symptoms or events occurring during sleep?

Clarify the presence of any respiratory symptoms:
- Snoring
- Apnoeas
- Gasping or choking in sleep
- An inspiratory noise as opposed to the expiratory noise, i.e. inspiratory stridor (suggests vocal cord dysfunction)
- Catathrenia (episodes of deep inspiration followed by a long expiration associated with a groaning noise)
- Nocturnal wheezing
- Paroxysmal nocturnal dyspnoea—may indicate a cardiac cause
- Acid taste in mouth—may point towards gastro-oesophageal reflux
- Ask about daytime or other symptoms consistent with sleep apnoea:
  - Dry mouth or sore throat on waking
  - Early morning headache
  - History of recent weight gain
  - Nocturia
- In targeted history taking, ask about comorbidities often seen in association with OSA:
  - Hypertension
  - Type 2 diabetes mellitus (T2D)
  - Atrial fibrillation
  - Nocturnal cardiac arrhythmias.

Ask about abnormal movements during sleep:
- Kicking or twitching at night, especially the lower limbs, raises the possibility of PLMD, and should precipitate further questions regarding the presence of RLS:
  - Urge to move limbs, especially legs, often associated with sensory symptoms

- The urge has a circadian pattern, worse in the evening or night
- The urge is improved, sometimes transiently, by movement of affected body parts
- Immobility worsens the urge to move
- If the patient exhibits unusual behaviours such as shouting out, talking, or lashing out, obtain more details:
  - What time of night does this happen? Events in the first half of the night suggest a disorder arising from NREM sleep, while events happening in the latter half are more indicative of a REM phenomenon
  - How often do these events happen? NREM parasomnias typically occur once or twice a night, while REM parasomnias or epileptic phenomena often occur several times per night
  - Age of onset—NREM parasomnias often start in childhood and it is less usual for these conditions to start in older age
  - Are the events very similar each time? Highly stereotyped events point towards epilepsy
  - Does the patient get out of bed or interact with the environment? Both of these suggest a NREM parasomnia
  - Is any speech fully formed and intelligible, or is it simply mumbling or shouting?
  - Are these events associated with dream recall? If so, are the dreams of a narrative structure, or simply visual imagery?
  - Ask about night-time eating, sexual behaviour, emotional content, and recall of events
  - Is the patient confused when woken? This suggests a confusional arousal as part of a NREM phenomenon, or epilepsy
  - Has there been self-injury or injury to the bed partner?

Explore experiences surrounding the transition between wake and sleep:
- Does the patient exhibit repetitive movements when drifting off to sleep, suggesting rhythmic movement disorder?
- Is there reported sleep paralysis or hallucinations at sleep onset or offset, perhaps indicating narcolepsy?

Consider other diagnoses:
- Is there evidence of tooth grinding (bruxism), such as jaw pain on waking, wearing of teeth, or reports from the bed partner?
- Does the patient experience painful leg cramps?

Is the predominant picture one of excessive daytime sleepiness or long sleep duration?

In the first instance, it is important to ascertain that the patient is complaining of sleepiness rather than fatigue or tiredness. Sleepiness is an excessive tendency to fall asleep or feel drowsy, whereas tiredness/fatigue is generally felt in the whole body and is characterized by low energy levels. Fatigue is relieved by rest and inactivity, but the same rest and inactivity will usually make drowsiness worse. Sleeping may or may not help tiredness, and indeed many patients with fatigue will often complain of unrefreshing sleep, leading to referral to the sleep clinic. Memory complaints and concentration difficulties are common to both fatigue and excessive daytime sleepiness.

Fatigued or tired individuals are not productive, but to a large extent remain alert to their surroundings. In contrast, sleepiness/drowsiness affects alertness, concentration, and reaction times and is potentially hazardous. Drowsiness immediately precedes sleep onset following which the individual loses control. As a result, in safety-critical situations, sleepiness can be more dangerous than tiredness. Making this distinction is also important in diagnostic formulation, in selection of investigations, and in the management priorities.

Common causes of fatigue include:
- Anaemia
- Malignancy
- Chronic infections/inflammation
- Diabetes
- Chronic kidney disease
- Hypothyroidism
- Depression
- Chronic fatigue syndrome
- Drugs such as cytotoxics, beta blockers, etc.

This, of course, is not an exhaustive list. It is important to exclude the medical causes of fatigue before embarking on investigations to look for sleep-related causes such as sleep apnoea and RLS/periodic limb movements of sleep (PLMS) unless the history is suggestive.

A useful and well-validated tool to estimate the propensity to fall asleep in various situations is the Epworth Sleepiness Scale (Box. 2.1), but other features strongly pointing towards excessive sleepiness include:
- Daytime naps
- Irresistible sleep attacks, particularly in active situations
- Automatic behaviours, e.g. skipping paragraphs while reading, or finding that they have written nonsensical text in the middle of a piece of work.

Box 2.1 Epworth Sleepiness Scale

How likely are you to doze off or fall asleep in the following situations, in contrast to just feeling tired? This refers to your usual life in recent times. Even if you have not done some of these things recently, try to work out how they would have affected you. Use the following scale to choose the most appropriate number for each situation:

0 = would never doze
1 = slight chance of dozing
2 = moderate chance of dozing
3 = high chance of dozing

Situation	Chance of dozing
Sitting and reading	☐
Watching TV	☐
Sitting, inactive in a public place (e.g. a theatre or a meeting)	☐
As a passenger in a car for an hour without a break	☐
Lying down to rest in the afternoon when circumstances permit	☐
Sitting and talking to someone	☐
Sitting quietly after a lunch without alcohol	☐
In a car, while stopped for a few minutes in traffic	☐
Total (normal 10 or less)	☐

The commonest cause of excessive sleepiness is chronic sleep restriction, termed behaviourally induced insufficient sleep syndrome (BIISS). Therefore, the first step is to ascertain whether the patient has a sufficient sleep opportunity. If they do not, clarify why this is the case.

If BIISS is considered as a likely diagnosis, the patient should be given sleep hygiene advice, be asked to extend sleep opportunity to a sufficient duration (>8 hours), and be reassessed.

The next step is to look for features of any organic sleep disorder or medical problem that might cause daytime sleepiness:

- OSA (see earlier in topic)
- RLS or PLMD
- Circadian rhythm disorder
- Patients with NREM parasomnias as well as REM parasomnias may sometimes experience unrefreshing sleep
- Prescribed medications (➜ Chapter 28) or recreational/illicit drug use should be looked at as these may cause daytime sleepiness
- Medical issues such as hypothyroidism, haemochromatosis, or autoimmune disorders should be excluded as a cause of symptoms
- Psychiatric disorders, especially atypical depression.

If these causes have been explored, then consider if there are features of a hypersomnia of central origin:

- Narcolepsy is suggested by features such as brief, refreshing daytime naps, sleep paralysis, hypnogogic hallucinations, vivid dreaming, especially in brief daytime naps, and fragmented night-time sleep, and is almost confirmed by the presence of cataplexy—the sudden loss of muscle tone often triggered by strong emotion (➜ Chapter 14). Patients with this condition may also describe REM sleep behaviour disorder (➜ Chapter 18). Additional features of narcolepsy include sleep attacks while standing or eating, and onset after infection or vaccination
- Idiopathic hypersomnia (IH) should be considered in patients with a very long sleep time, consistently unrefreshing sleep, marked sleep inertia or drunkenness, and long unrefreshing daytime naps
- Recurrent episodes of excessive sleepiness with behavioural change are a feature of Kleine–Levin syndrome.

It is also important to understand the impact of EDS on other aspects of the patient's life:

- Driving (➜ Chapter 29), and operating heavy machinery
- Ability to engage in work, education, and social life.

Useful clinical tools

A number of questionnaires are available which can help in the evaluation of patients with sleep disorders. The Epworth Sleepiness Scale (➲ Box. 2.1, p. 16), is one of the most commonly used in clinical practice and provides a measure of sleepiness over the last few weeks. Other helpful questionnaires include:
- Stanford Sleepiness Scale, which measures sleepiness at a particular point
- Pittsburgh Sleep Quality Index, a general questionnaire
- Sleep diaries/questionnaires
- Berlin Questionnaire, which screens for OSA
- Functional Outcomes of Sleep Questionnaire (FOSQ)
- Sleep Apnoea Quality of Life Index (SAQLI)
- Beck Depression Inventory (BDI).

Clinical decision-making in sleep medicine

Many patients referred to sleep clinics will not require extensive and expensive investigations, or expensive medications. Most will benefit from basic sleep hygiene advice. In fact, the first treatment step in all sleep disorders should be sleep hygiene advice.

After reviewing the history and examining the patient, a decision will then have to be made as to which investigations should be carried out (➔ Chapter 3) or which treatment should be offered.

Findings of particular concern include the following:

- Hypersomnolence:
  - Dangerous sleepiness which needs immediate attention as manifested by repeated sleep attacks—this could be due to a condition such as sleep apnoea or central hypersomnolence
  - Significant cardiac risk if associated with sleep-disordered breathing (SDB)
  - If the patient is a professional driver or is in any other safety-critical occupation
- Parasomnias:
  - History of violent behaviours or injury to self or others during sleep, or risk thereof
  - Frequent sleepwalking or other out-of-bed behaviour
  - New onset of uncharacteristic sleep behaviours
  - The need to exclude other serious pathology such as epilepsy
- Insomnia:
  - Debilitating insomnia with impairment of daytime functionality.

Other reasons for referral include the severity of effects on the patient's (or bed partner's) life, such as:

- Daytime functioning
- Academic, social, and workplace functioning
- Relationships with partner or other family members
- Patient's other health outcomes, e.g. cardiovascular morbidity
- Impact on the bed partner or other family members
- Disturbed night-time sleep (from loud snoring, partner's restless sleep).

These symptoms will also inform treatment decisions.

Conclusion

- A basic understanding of normal sleep is essential
- Identification of a possible sleep disorder through history taking is the initial first step
- Evaluation of the symptoms of the entire 24-hour period should be made
- The sleep–wake patterns should be noted
- Additional history from the partner should be obtained
- An attempt to define the specific sleep problem should then be made
- Evaluation of the impact of the disorder on the patient and their partner/family is the next step
- Once the initial evaluation is complete, the clinician may generate a differential diagnosis
- On the basis of relative likelihood of diagnostic possibilities, appropriate diagnostic studies may be carried out
- Even when the diagnosis is clear, laboratory tests may be required to determine the severity of the condition
- Appropriate treatment will then follow.

Further reading

Kushida CA, Littner MR, Morgenthaler T, et al. Practice parameters for the indications for polysomnography and related procedures: an update for 2005. Sleep. 2005;28(4):499–521.

Sateia MJ. International classification of sleep disorders–third edition: highlights and modifications. Chest. 2014;146(5):1387–94.

Sateia MJ, Thorpy MJ. Classification of sleep disorders. In: Kryger MH, Roth T, Dement WC (Eds) Principles and Practice of Sleep Medicine, 6th ed. Philadelphia, PA: Elsevier; 2015:618–26.

Silber MH. Diagnostic approach and investigation in sleep medicine. Continuum (Minneap Minn). 2017;23(4):973–88.

Diagnostic tests in sleep medicine

Seán E. Higgins

Introduction

A wide variety of diagnostic tests exist to aid the clinician in diagnosing sleep disorders. These range from simple and relatively cheap home diagnostic tests such as pulse oximetry to in-laboratory video polysomnography (vPSG), which is expensive and labour intensive. Understanding the indications for and limitations of these diagnostic tests allows the accurate diagnosis of sleep disorders in a timely manner, while best managing limited resources. Diagnostic tests should be interpreted by trained, suitably qualified personnel and used to complement conventional clinical practice and decision-making.

Pulse oximetry

Pulse oximetry is a simple non-invasive method for assessing arterial oxygen saturation. Oximeters emit two known wavelengths of light and measure its absorption, thus calculating oxygen saturation. Devices used for sleep recordings take a minimum of one sample per second and average the readings over a 3-second rolling window. The data is stored in the device and can easily be downloaded to a computer for analysis.

- Pulse oximetry can be used as a screening test for OSA in patients who have a high pretest probability
- The 4% oxygen desaturation index (ODI) broadly reflects the apnoea–hypopnoea index (AHI), the gold standard for assessing severity of sleep apnoea, but unlike the AHI does not require airflow or EEG channels.
  - 4% ODI 5–15 indicates mild sleep apnoea
  - 4% ODI 16–30 indicates moderate sleep apnoea
  - 4% ODI >30 indicates severe sleep apnoea
- Test reliability can be improved by performing the test on two consecutive nights
- Negative results may simply reflect lack of sleep on the night of the test
- Pulse oximetry will not detect clinically significant upper airway resistance syndrome (UARS), which requires EEG channels to assess for arousals related to respiratory events
- Patients with a high clinical suspicion for OSA with negative pulse oximetry results should be investigated further with either polygraphy or PSG studies.

Respiratory polygraphy studies

Respiratory polygraphy can be used in the hospital or home setting to screen patients for OSA. A wide variety of devices are available for performing respiratory polygraphy studies. Some variance exists between devices but typically each device will record:

- Pulse oximetry
- Airflow:
  - From nasal pressure swings, or
  - From oronasal thermistor
- Snoring
- Respiratory effort—some devices use a single effort sensor whereas others separately measure thoracic and abdominal effort
- Body position—useful to identify position-dependent sleep apnoea
- Devices utilizing peripheral arterial tonometry rather than airflow and respiratory effort can also be used and provide added simplicity for the patient.

As with simple pulse oximetry, these respiratory polygraphy studies do not measure sleep and negative test results may require more detailed investigation.

Video polysomnography

vPSG is the 'gold standard' test for investigating sleep disorders. It may be performed as an unattended home test but is typically performed under direct supervision in the sleep laboratory. vPSG requires trained personnel to prepare the patient for the test, to supervise the test, and to analyse and report the findings (Fig. 3.1).

Each study will typically record:
- Electro-oculogram (EOG):
  - Slow rolling eye movements during drowsiness and at sleep onset
  - Rapid eye movements during REM sleep
- EEG:
  - Distinguishes wake from NREM and REM sleep
  - Typically, six channels are used but a full 10–20 montage may be used when investigating patients with epilepsy
- Electromyogram (EMG):
  - EMG tone diminished during REM sleep
  - Identifies pathologies such as bruxism, periodic limb movements, and loss of REM atonia
- ECG to identify arrhythmias
- The parameters mentioned in the respiratory polygraphy section:
  - Distinguishes central sleep apnoea (CSA) from OSA
  - Identifies flow limitation events
  - May include carbon dioxide (CO_2) monitoring to identify hypoventilation in sleep
- The study includes audio and video which is time-locked to the physiological signals. This is invaluable when investigating:
  - Slow-wave parasomnias
  - Rhythmic movement disorder
  - Sleep-related hypermotor epilepsy.

vPSG is recommended for the investigation of:
- *Narcolepsy*: vPSG (with multiple sleep latency test (MSLT; see later in this chapter) performed the following day) is indicated in the evaluation of suspected narcolepsy
- *Nocturnal seizures*: vPSG with extended montage EEG is indicated when clinical evaluation and standard EEG is inconclusive
- *Parasomnias*: vPSG is indicated in atypical or unusual sleep behaviours and can differentiate between non-REM parasomnias and REM-related parasomnias
- *Violent sleep behaviours*: vPSG with extended montage EEG and digital video is indicated (e.g. REM sleep behaviour disorder (RBD), sleepwalking, forensic cases)
- *Periodic limb movement disorder (PLMD)*.

vPSG is *not* recommended for the investigation of:
- Circadian rhythm disorders
- Depression
- RLS
- Insomnia, unless other sleep disorders are suspected.

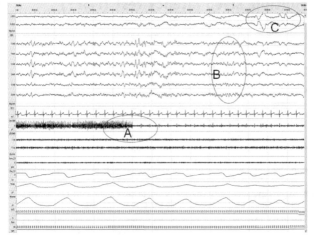

Fig. 3.1 A 30-second 'epoch' from a polysomnography study showing the transition from N2 sleep to REM sleep. Note the loss of muscle tone in submental EMG at A, 'sawtooth waves' in the EEG at B, and rapid eye movements in the EOG traces at C.

Multiple sleep latency test (MSLT)

The MSLT is a test designed to objectively measure a patient's propensity to fall asleep. It is used primarily in the diagnosis of narcolepsy and central (idiopathic) hypersomnia.

The test records EOG, EEG, EMG, and ECG.

- The test consists of four or five 'nap' tests performed at 2-hourly intervals following a vPSG study
- Each test session allows a 20-minute window for the patient to fall asleep:
  - If sleep is reached, the test session terminates 15 minutes after sleep onset
  - Patients must remain awake between test sessions
- A mean sleep latency (MSL) of <8 minutes and two sleep-onset REM periods is considered positive for narcolepsy
- An MSL of <8 minutes without sleep-onset REM periods may indicate a primary hypersomnia
- Trained personnel are required to be present during the test as sleep staging must be performed while the test in progress.

The MSLT may be strongly influenced by prior sleep and medication (e.g. REM-suppressing antidepressants) and may yield both false-positive and false-negative results.

Maintenance of wakefulness test (MWT)

The MWT is a test designed to determine a subject's ability to maintain wakefulness in a non-stimulating environment. Parameters recorded are similar to the MSLT, but the test is performed with the patient sitting re-clined on a bed in a dimly lit room. Four 40-minute tests are performed at 2-hourly intervals.

The subject is asked to:
- Sit quietly on the bed
- Keep their eyes open and try to remain awake
- Fidgeting or other forms of distraction are not permitted.

Each session is terminated:
- After 40 minutes if the patient manages to remain awake
- After three consecutive epochs (one epoch = 30 seconds) of N1 sleep, or
- Any epoch of another sleep stage.

In the UK, the MWT *may* be performed when patients need evidence to support their application for return of a driving licence. The MWT test re-sult can only *support* clinical judgement as:
- There is a wide range of normal results
- No firm consensus exists as to what defines a failure of the MWT
- The test does not directly measure the subject's ability to remain awake and alert behind the wheel.

Oxford Sleep Resistance Test (OSLER)

The OSLER is a test designed to mimic the MWT test but is simpler to perform and administer. No recording electrodes are required.

- Four 40-minute test sessions are performed at 2-hourly intervals
- The subject is seated reclined on a bed in a dimly lit room
- The subject is required to press a button in response to a dim red light which flashes once every 3 seconds
- Seven consecutive misses are considered to represent sleep, at which point the test terminates
- The total number of misses over the whole of the test session may relate to the subject's level of vigilance
- Some groups suggest shorter (20-minute) tests are adequate and others that fewer than four tests are adequate, but a consensus does not exist
- An advantage of the OSLER is that it can be performed in a setting where PSG is unavailable
- As with the MWT, the OSLER test does not directly measure the subject's ability to remain awake and alert behind the wheel.

Actigraphy

Actigraphy consists of a small device (similar to a wrist watch) which uses an accelerometer to measure and record movement. The devices can be used to record over a prolonged period and can give a useful picture of a patient's sleep patterns (Fig. 3.2). It is widely used in sleep research and in the clinical sleep setting.

- Actigraphy is recommended for the investigation of circadian rhythm disorders, e.g.:
  - Advanced sleep phase syndrome
  - Delayed sleep phase syndrome
  - Shift work disorder
  - Non-24-hour sleep/wake syndrome
- It is increasingly also being used in clinical practice to evaluate sleep/ wake patterns in patients for a period of weeks prior to MSLT testing
- Actigraphy measures movement, and may underestimate sleep in some individuals and overestimate in others
- Additional software-derived parameters such as fragmentation indices are not alternatives to a PSG-derived arousal index and should be interpreted with caution
- Actigraphy can provide a useful measure when determining response to treatment in patients with circadian rhythm disorders
- The advice in this section refers only to properly validated actigraphy devices. A growing number of non-validated commercial devices are available, and are actively marketed to the public. Information from these devices should treated with great caution and is not equivalent to validated actigraphy.

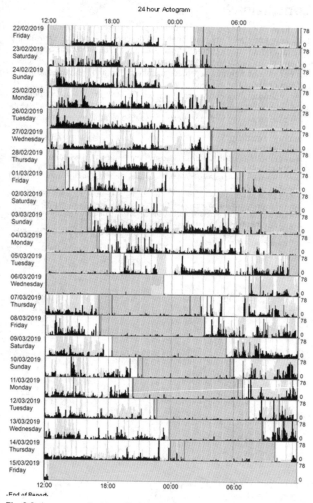

Fig. 3.2 An actogram (activity in black, light levels in yellow and sleep phase shaded) from a 21-day study showing a non-24-hour circadian rhythm with sleep phase shifting on a daily basis.

Conclusion

The diagnostic tests described in this chapter are well-validated tests whose sensitivity and specificity have been well described. A host of devices and smartphone apps are currently marketed to the public which purport to monitor sleep depth and quality. The accuracy of such devices has generally not been verified against accepted gold standards, and their use in the clinical setting should be avoided.

Appropriate diagnostic testing should be undertaken—and their results interpreted—in the context of the overall clinical picture. These tests should be requested with a view to providing a clinically relevant answer.

Further reading

Hirshkowitz M. Polysomnography and beyond. In: Kryger MH, Roth T, Dement WC (Eds) Principles and Practice of Sleep Medicine, 6th ed. Philadelphia, PA: Elsevier; 2017:1564–66.

Kapur V, Auckley DH, Chowdhuri S, et al. Clinical practice guideline for diagnostic testing for adult obstructive sleep apnea: an American Academy of Sleep Medicine Clinical Practice Guideline. J Clin Sleep Med. 2017;13(3):479–504.

Kushida C, Littner MR, Morgenthaler T, et al. Practice parameters for the indications for polysomnography and related procedures: an update for 2005. Sleep. 2005;28(4):499–521.

Littner MR, Kushida C, Wise M, et al. Practice parameters for clinical use of the multiple sleep latency test and the Maintenance of Wakefulness Test. Sleep. 2005;28(1):113–21.

Penzel T (2017). Home sleep testing. In Principles and Practice of Sleep Medicine, 6th ed. Philadelphia, PA: Elsevier Inc; 2017: 610–1614.

Clinical aspects of insomnia

Hugh Selsick and *David O'Regan*

Introduction

Insomnia is the most common sleep disorder, and frequently coexists with other medical, psychiatric, and sleep conditions. It is associated with significant personal and socioeconomic burdens. The clinical features, assessment, epidemiology, consequences of insomnia, diagnosis, differential diagnosis, and treatment are discussed here. The pharmacological and non-pharmacological treatments of insomnia are discussed in more detail in ➔ Chapters 5 and 6.

What is insomnia?

Insomnia is:
- Persistent difficulty in falling asleep, and/or
- Persistent difficulty in remaining asleep for a sufficient period of time, and/or
- Persistent inability to have consolidated sleep
- Which occurs despite having adequate sleep opportunity, and
- Leads to daytime dysfunction, and
- Is not better explained by another sleep disorder.

It is important to note that:
- Short sleep in the absence of daytime dysfunction or distress does not constitute insomnia. These people are simply short sleepers and it does not constitute a sleep disorder
- Short sleep due to inadequate sleep opportunity is not insomnia. This is insufficient sleep syndrome, also known as sleep restriction or sleep deprivation. The effects and treatment of this disorder is very different to that of insomnia.

Diagnostic categories
- Chronic insomnia: symptoms occur at least three times a week for at least 3 months
- Short-term insomnia disorder: symptoms last <3 months
- Other insomnia disorder: insomnia symptoms that do not meet criteria for chronic or short-term insomnia.

Subtypes

Although there are numerous subtypes of insomnia, the concept of primary and secondary insomnias has fallen out of favour and all insomnia should be addressed, regardless of the subtype or the comorbidities. However, sometimes identifying a particular subtype can be helpful in identifying the focus of therapeutic interventions:
- Insomnia can be associated with other medical disorders, medications, and other substances or mental disorders
- Psychophysiological insomnia—where there are learned associations that prevent sleep, heightened arousal, and excessive anxiety about sleep
- Inadequate sleep hygiene—where the patient has dysfunctional sleep-related behaviours
- Behavioural insomnia of childhood—where the child's sleep training or the parents' limit-setting was inadequate
- Paradoxical insomnia is the complaint of significant sleep disturbance which is not confirmed on objective studies. Some of the time when they are asleep, patients subjectively feel they are awake. Many patients with genuine insomnia have an element of this sleep state misperception and will underestimate their actual sleep duration.

Epidemiology

Prevalence rates

Studies on the prevalence of insomnia have been hampered by variations in case definitions, assessment procedures, sample characteristics, and assessment period length. As a result, published prevalence rates vary from 5% to 50%.

- At least 33% of adult populations report one nocturnal insomnia symptom
- This drops to 10–15% when daytime symptoms (e.g. tiredness) are included
- When using diagnostic criteria (e.g. International Classification of Sleep Disorders, third edition), prevalence rates vary between 6% and 10%:
  - The removal of the non-specific symptom 'non-restorative sleep' from the newer diagnostic manuals may in part account for this reduction.

Prevalence rates are consistently higher among:
- Women (risk ratio of 1.41:1)
- Middle-aged and older adults
- Shift workers
- Patients with comorbid physical and mental health disorders (odds ratio of 4.0–6.0)
- Patients of lower socioeconomic status
- Patients who live alone (e.g. single, separated, or widowed).

The role of ethnicity and culture

Ethnicity and culture also affect prevalence rates. People from different cultures experience and perceive health problems differently (e.g. as a result of religious beliefs, stigma, and symptom presentation).

In a nationwide sleep survey in the US, insomnia was diagnosed in:
- 10% of whites
- 7% of Hispanics
- 4% of Asians
- 3% of African Americans.

A worldwide study of insomnia found the highest prevalence of insomnia in:
- Brazil (~79%)
- South Africa (~45%)
- Eastern Europe (32%)
- Asia (28%)
- Western Europe (~23%).

Risk factors

The most commonly hypothesized predisposing factors for insomnia include:

- Female sex (especially at menopause)
- First-degree family members of individuals with insomnia. It is unclear if this is genetically mediated, *or* is secondary to learned behaviours, *or* is a by-product of other disorders (e.g. mental health illness)
- A past personal history of insomnia
- Psychological vulnerability (e.g. anxiety-prone personality)
- Biological vulnerability (e.g. increased hypothalamic–pituitary–adrenal axis activity).

Trajectory of insomnia

Insomnia is often persistent over time. Depending on the interval between assessments, persistence rates vary significantly:

- In the Cardiovascular Health Study, persistent rates of insomnia over a 1-year to 4-year period were:
  - 15.4% for difficulty in falling asleep
  - 22.7% for difficulty with sleep maintenance
- Most studies choose an interval period of 1 year, which may underestimate the fluctuating nature of insomnia. For example, when individuals were assessed on a monthly basis, one study showed that 69% of participants changed their sleeping status at least once over a 12-month period. So, an individual with insomnia at baseline, may recover at 6 months, and relapse again by 12 months
- Factors associated with persistence of insomnia include:
  - Female sex
  - Older age
  - Medical problems
  - Mental health illnesses.

Consequences of insomnia

Short-term consequences of insomnia

The short-term consequences of insomnia are significant, distressing, and negatively impact every aspect of life. They are often the driving force for a person with insomnia seeking help. They include daily:
- Fatigue
- Tiredness
- Unpleasant body sensations (e.g. heavy eyes)
- Perceptual hypersensitivity (e.g. to noise, light)
- Mood disturbance (e.g. irritability, increased emotional reactivity)
- Negative personal interactions (e.g. with children, partners)
- Reduced self-esteem, optimism, and confidence
- Poor quality of life
- Feeling alone and misunderstood
- Cognitive disturbance (e.g. reduced attention, concentration, performance).

Long-term consequences of insomnia

Psychological health

Insomnia is strongly associated with poor mental health, and is an important risk factor for the development of mental health disorders.

Chronic insomnia is associated with:
- Two times higher risk of future anxiety
- Four times higher risk of future depression
- Increased risk of suicide intentions, attempts, and successes.

These higher risks have been demonstrated in children, adolescents, and adults, and are independent of past personal and family history of other mental health disorders.

The relationship between insomnia and mental health disorders is bidirectional, i.e. insomnia may be the cause or the result of a mental health disorder:
- Insomnia negatively impacts the trajectory of mental health illnesses. For example, depressed patients with insomnia have significantly poorer outcomes, with respect to symptom ratings, attrition and remission rates, and stability of response to treatment when compared to depressed patients without insomnia
- Insomnia is an independent risk factor for the development of schizophrenia, and exacerbates psychotic experiences. Up to 44% of patients with schizophreniform disorders have a comorbid insomnia, which is independently associated with reduced quality of life
- In bipolar affective disorder (BPAD), insomnia frequently triggers manic episodes, and becomes more severe as the mania unfolds. Between episodes, up to 70% of patients experience difficulties with insomnia, which further negatively impacts mood and daytime functioning
- Sleep difficulties go hand in hand with post-traumatic stress disorder (PTSD). In patients who have otherwise achieved remission, debilitating insomnia often persists.
- In alcohol dependence, up to 72% of patients who achieve abstinence experience chronic insomnia. The residual insomnia is often a significant relapse factor.

Physical health

The link between insomnia and physical health disorders is not as well defined:

- Many studies demonstrating an association between insomnia and physical health disorders have been criticized for their small patient numbers and lack of appropriate investigations to exclude other sleep disorders (e.g. SDB)
- Overcoming these barriers, epidemiological studies from the Penn State Adult Cohort objectively examined insomnia using PSG. An emerging distinction appears between patients with chronic insomnia who experience physiological hyperarousal, and those who experience cognitive-emotional arousal, i.e.:
  - Physiological hyperarousal—sleep of short duration (≤6 hours) associated with activation of the stress system
  - Cognitive-emotional arousal—sleep of normal duration (≥6 hours) associated with normal activity of the stress system
- Chronic insomnia associated with physiological hyperarousal appears to be associated with significant physical health sequelae, whereas chronic insomnia associated with cognitive-emotional arousal does not (Table 4.1).

Table 4.1 Physical health sequelae associated with chronic insomnia

Sequelae	Sleep of short duration	Sleep of normal duration
Physiological hyperarousal, i.e.:	√	X
Increased cortisol levels	√	X
Increased heart rate variability	√	X
Increased metabolic rate	√	X
Increased daytime alertness	√	X
Hypertension	√ (5.1)	X (1.3)
Diabetes	√ (2.95)	X (1.1)
Mortality (men only)	√ (4.0)	X

√ denotes association; X denotes non-association. Odds ratios are shown in brackets. Sleep of short duration defined as sleep of ≤6 hours. Sleep of normal duration defined as sleep ≥6 hours.

Occupational health

The daytime dysfunction associated with insomnia particularly affects the workplace. It is recognized as significant barrier in the achievement of personal career goals.

Chronic insomnia is associated with:
- Reduced productivity
- Absenteeism
- Being late for work
- Reduced professional advancement (e.g. promotion, salary increase)
- Reduced job satisfaction
- Reduced coping skills—particularly in problem-solving
- Lower feelings of mastery
- Increased intentions of switching occupations
- Permanent work disability
- Increased risk of personal and work-related errors and accidents (*not* motor vehicle-related accidents).

Economic consequences

Insomnia carries very significant direct and indirect economic costs for society:
- Direct costs include insomnia-related medical consultations, transport to and from clinics, prescriptions, over-the-counter medications, and alcohol used as a sleep aid
- Indirect costs include work absenteeism and insomnia-related reduced productivity
- In the US, insomnia is estimated to cost between $63 and $90 billion per year, with one study showing 75% of the burden being related to its indirect costs
- The cost of insomnia has not been calculated in the UK, though one study reported that reduced sleep (defined as regularly sleeping ≤6 hours per night) cost the economy £40 billion per year
- Insomnia severity and frequency show a dose–response effect with direct healthcare costs. For example, in the US, individuals with moderate to severe insomnia can pay double the cost of medical insurance when compared to good sleepers
- Indirectly, insomnia severity also shows a dose–response curve for reduced productivity costs, e.g. an employee with insomnia disorder has indirect employment more than four times that of an employee with insomnia symptoms, and more than 12 times that of an employee without insomnia.

Diagnosis

In the majority of cases, the diagnosis of insomnia is made on the history; investigations are occasionally required, but they are usually to exclude any other sleep disorders that may be suspected from the history.

History

The history should achieve the following goals:
- Determine if the patient meets diagnostic criteria for insomnia
- Ascertain any precipitating factors for the insomnia
- Ascertain any perpetuating factors for the insomnia
- Detect or exclude any comorbid sleep, medical, or psychiatric disorders that may be mimicking or exacerbating the insomnia.

Does the patient meet criteria for insomnia?

Ask the patient to describe a typical night's sleep including the times they go to bed and rise. This is also an opportunity to determine if there are any dysfunctional behaviours and cognitions that perpetuate the insomnia:
- Do they have difficulty initiating sleep?
- Do they have fragmented sleep?
- Do they have long periods of wakefulness in the night?
- Do they have early morning waking?
- How much sleep do they think they are getting?
- What do they do before bed?
- What do they do when they first get into bed?
- What do they do during periods of wakefulness in the night?

Determine how frequently they sleep badly and for how long they have had the symptoms:
- How many nights a week does this happen? Does it occur at least 3 nights a week? This will also allow you to determine if there is any pattern to the insomnia. For example, are there specific nights of the week where they sleep better or worse and why is this?
- How long have they had the symptoms; has it been longer than 3 months?
- Have the symptoms gotten worse with time, do they fluctuate, or is there a seasonal element to them?

Determine how their sleep affects them during the day:
- Does it cause fatigue?
- Are there any cognitive consequences?
- Does it impact their mood, irritability, etc.?
- Does it impact their relationships?
- How does it affect their work?
- Are there any safety issues (e.g. car accidents due to fatigue)?

Precipitating factors for insomnia

There are innumerable precipitating factors for insomnia. Stress, environmental factors, depression, anxiety disorders, substance misuse, pain, illness, medications, and pregnancy are but a few. If the precipitating factor is still present, then it may indicate the insomnia may recover once the precipitant is removed and the treatment will be focused on managing the insomnia until the precipitating factor resolves. However, in chronic insomnia, the precipitant will usually have resolved by the time the patient seeks medical help. In this case, the precipitant has relatively little relevance for the treatment of the insomnia, but patients often appreciate having the opportunity to explain how their insomnia started.

Perpetuating factors for insomnia

Insomnia can be perpetuated by dysfunctional habits and cognitions such as:

• Excessive focus on, and ruminations about, sleep
• Reducing the homeostatic sleep drive by going to bed too early, sleeping too late in the morning, or having variable rising times and napping (intentionally or unintentionally) during the day
• Watching television or using phones in bed, etc. and spending time in the bedroom during the day. This develops an association between the bed/bedroom and wakefulness rather than with sleep
• Incorrect use of sleeping medications or stimulants
• Avoiding activities during the day due to concerns about ability to function when tired
• Learned anxiety about sleep. This often manifests as gradually increasing anxiety before bedtime, or once in bed.

Ascertaining these perpetuating factors allows you to devise a treatment plan that addresses these factors.

Detecting or excluding other sleep disorders

Almost any other sleep disorder could exacerbate insomnia and some can mimic insomnia. In particular, one should look for:

• RLS: it is surprising how few patients with restless legs volunteer this symptom. They will usually present with a complaint of difficulty initiating and, sometimes, maintaining sleep. It is therefore essential to ask all insomnia patients about restless legs
• Nightmares, sleep terrors, and other parasomnias: some patients develop a fear of sleeping because they are anxious about having a parasomnia episode
• OSA: although this more commonly presents with excessive sleepiness, it not infrequently causes insomnia instead
• Circadian rhythm disorders: these should be suspected if the timing of sleep and of alertness is unusual but the sleep, once initiated, is normal in all other respects.

Excessive sleepiness during the day can be a symptom of uncomplicated insomnia but, as the majority of insomnia patients are 'tired but wired', daytime sleepiness should raise the suspicion that there may be an organic sleep disorder as well

Sleep diaries and scales

While there are a number of scales that examine insomnia symptoms, they are more useful in audit and research than in clinical settings. The Insomnia Severity Index (ISI) is a well-validated and widely used scale which can be useful for monitoring a patient's response to treatment. The Epworth Sleepiness Scale (→ Box 2.1, p. 16) can also be helpful to determine if there is excessive daytime sleepiness, which may mitigate for an organic sleep disorder or have safety implications.

Much more useful are sleep diaries. When asked to describe their sleep, patients will often give the worst-case scenario and they may have difficulty explaining the night-to-night variability in their sleep. A sleep diary provides a longitudinal picture of their sleep, which is also helpful in picking out patterns and perpetuating factors.

Investigations

Medical investigations are rarely needed in insomnia unless there is a clinical suspicion of another sleep disorder or underlying medical disorder. Investigations one may consider include:

- Thyroid function
- Ferritin, folate, vitamin B_{12}, kidney function, and blood sugar if you suspect restless legs or periodic limb movements
- Full blood count if you suspect infection or anaemia as a cause of the fatigue
- ECG if you are going to prescribe any medications which may prolong the QTc interval.

Actigraphy can be useful if the patient is a poor historian or cannot keep a sleep diary. It may also be helpful to confirm a suspicion of a circadian rhythm disorder.

PSG may be considered in the following cases:

- If you suspect another sleep disorder such as periodic limb movements, parasomnias, or OSA
- If the patient presents with paradoxical insomnia. The PSG can be very reassuring to the patient when they see that they are getting some sleep, or more sleep than they realized
- If a patient has not responded to standard insomnia treatments.

Treatment

- If there is a precipitating factor, such as pain, anxiety, or alerting medication, then treat that factor
- However, do not assume that treating the precipitant will always cure the insomnia—often insomnia will persist after the precipitant has resolved
- Therefore, one should treat the insomnia assertively as well
- Treatment may involve hypnotics or psychological and behavioural interventions. These are discussed in more detail in ➜ Chapters 5 and 6.

Further reading

American Academy of Sleep Medicine. International Classification of Sleep Disorders, 3rd ed. Darien, IL: American Academy of Sleep Medicine; 2014.

Fernandez-Mendoza J. The insomnia with short sleep duration phenotype: an update on its import-ance for health and prevention. Curr Opin Psychiatry. 2017;30(1):56–63.

Fernandez-Mendoza J, Vgontzas AN, Liao D, et al. Insomnia with objective short sleep duration and incident hypertension: the Penn State Cohort. Hypertension. 2012;60(4):929–35.

Morin CM, Jarrin DC. Epidemiology of insomnia. Sleep Med Clin. 2013;8(3):281–97.

Selsick H. Insomnia assessment. In: Selsick H (Ed) Sleep Disorders in Psychiatric Patients: A Practical Guide. Berlin: Springer; 2018:109–19.

Wilson SJ, Nutt DJ, Alford C, et al. British Association for Psychopharmacology consensus state-ment on evidence-based treatment of insomnia, parasomnias and circadian rhythm disorders. J Psychopharmacol. 2010;24(11):1577–601.

Chapter 5

Psychological therapies for insomnia

David O'Regan

Introduction

Insomnia is defined as difficulty in initiating or maintaining sleep with associated impaired daytime functioning. It is the most common sleep and mental health disorder, present in ~10–30% of the adult population. The consequences of insomnia are significant, including increased risk of health problems, work absenteeism, reduced productivity, increased healthcare utilization, and non-motor-vehicle accidents.

Psychological and behavioural therapies are recommended as the first-line and gold standard treatments for insomnia. This chapter summarizes common non-pharmacological treatment approaches, as well as the evidence base supporting their use. Emerging treatment options are also outlined. Consideration is given to special populations, including older adults, children and teens, comorbid insomnia, and individuals taking hypnotics. Practical aspects of administering therapy are also summarized, including contraindications, risks, managing resistance, and relapse prevention.

Recommended psychological and behavioural therapies

The American Academy of Sleep Medicine (AASM) considers the following treatments as standard for insomnia:
- Stimulus control therapy
- Relaxation training
- Cognitive behavioural therapy for insomnia (CBT-I).

The following additional therapies have received some support by the AASM:
- Sleep restriction
- Multicomponent therapy without cognitive therapy
- Paradoxical intention
- Biofeedback approaches.

The following are not recommended as *stand-alone* therapies by the AASM:
- Sleep hygiene
- Imagery training
- Cognitive therapy.

Summary of treatment components

Treatment	Description
Stimulus control	Aims to restore the learned association between the bed/bedroom and sleeping. Patient is instructed only to go the bedroom for sleep, getting dressed, and sex. The patient is advised to leave the bed/bedroom if they are awake for 15 minutes, and to return again when they feel sleepy. Napping is discouraged, and regular wake and bed times are set.
Sleep restriction	Consists of limiting the amount of time spent in bed to the actual time spent sleeping. Achieved by setting a prescribed bed and wake time, which is subsequently adjusted according to the sleep efficiency (SE).
Sleep compression	A variation of sleep restriction where the time in bed is gradually reduced, typically in weekly 15-minute increments. Advised for patients where sleep restriction may exacerbate comorbid conditions (e.g. bipolar affective disorder, migraine, epilepsy, chronic fatigue syndrome, etc.).
Relaxation	Physical and mental techniques used to reduce hyperarousal. Examples include progressive muscular relaxation, guided imagery, and mediation.
Cognitive therapy	Uncovers sleep/insomnia myths, and provides alternate explanations. Allows the patient to reframe their insomnia.
CBT-I	A treatment package, which usually comprises sleep hygiene, stimulus control, sleep restriction, relaxation training, and cognitive therapy.

Outline of psychological and behavioural interventions

Stimulus control

- Effective monotherapy for insomnia based on classical conditioning
- For a good sleeper, the stimulus of the bed/bedroom acts as a cue to induce sleep
- Patients with insomnia often have a history of engaging in sleep-disrupting behaviours in the bedroom (e.g. watching TV, eating, worrying, reading, etc.)
- They perceive that spending more time in bed will increase their chances of getting more sleep
- These maladaptive behaviours actually weaken the stimulus–response relationship between being in bed and falling asleep
- Over time, the stimuli of the bed/bedroom become cues for anxiety and frustration with trying to fall asleep
- Instructions for stimulus control are outlined in ● Summary of treatment components, p. 47
- It is contraindicated for patients with comorbidities: epilepsy, parasomnias, mania, and those at risks of falls.

Sleep restriction

- Aims to limit the amount of time spent in bed to the actual time spent asleep
- Sleep diary data are used to establish the average times in bed and asleep from the previous 2 weeks
- SE is calculated by dividing the average time asleep by the average time in bed and multiplying this number by 100
- A good sleeper has a SE of ≥90%
- The patient's SE is used to determine the prescribed time in bed
- Usually, the patient will set an anchor time, i.e. the latest time they will get out of bed/bedroom each morning, 7 days a week, regardless of how well they have slept
- The average sleep time is subtracted from this anchor time in order to determine the sleep threshold, i.e. the earliest time they can go to bed, provided they are sleepy
- The minimum amount of time in bed is set to 5 hours, except in bipolar affective disorder, where it is set to 6 hours
- During subsequent weeks, the time in bed is up- or down-titrated depending on the SE
- This is usually achieved by altering the sleep threshold by 15 minutes, i.e.:
  - SE ≥90%: bring forward to earliest bedtime by 15 minutes
  - SE 85–89%: make no changes
  - SE <90%: delay the earliest bedtime by 15 minutes
- The technique allows the patient to accrue a small sleep debt, whereby they fall asleep more easily on subsequent nights, and their sleep becomes more consolidated
- An increase in daytime fatigue is a transient difficulty in the early stages
- It is contraindicated for patients with bipolar affective disorder, epilepsy, OSA, professional drivers, chronic fatigue syndrome, migraine, or any other condition where sleep loss will exacerbate their comorbid conditions.

Sleep compression

- A variation of sleep restriction, where the time in bed is gradually reduced
- Advised for patients where sleep restriction is contraindicated, or where anxiety of sleep restriction is overwhelming
- The patient agrees the latest bedtime acceptable to them, and each week this is delayed by 15 minutes until their SE reaches 90%.

Relaxation

- Reduces the pre-bed and in-bed mental and physical tension and hyperarousal that many patients with insomnia experience
- Examples include progressive muscular relaxation, guided imagery, mediation, and autogenic training. Autogenic training utilizes the body's natural relaxation response to counteract unwanted mental and physical symptoms via the use of breathing techniques, specific verbal stimuli, and mindful meditation
- Patients are encouraged to trial a variety of techniques and to use them in combination, e.g. commence with progressive muscular relaxation and, if needed, move to guided imagery
- It must be emphasized that these techniques take time to work, and practice is key.

Paradoxical intention

- The patient is instructed to follow their usual pre-bed routine
- They are then asked to focus on staying awake during the night
- By focusing on staying awake, the frustration and stress with trying to achieve sleep is relieved.

Cognitive therapy

- The patient's held myths regarding sleep are uncovered
- An alternate explanation is provided, allowing the patient to view their insomnia in a different way (see following 'Primary aims')
- Time for constructive worry is encouraged, as a means of 'putting the day to bed'. The patient writes down their worries and possible solutions for these. The aim is to empty the mind of worries before entering the bedroom
- Techniques to deal with worries in the night are also taught (e.g. thought stopping techniques).

Primary aims of cognitive therapy

Correcting misconceptions about the causes of insomnia

Patients often attribute insomnia as being out of their control, e.g. due to an external cause. However, insomnia always involves some psychological and behavioural factors that the patient can modify. Patients are encouraged to focus on these modifiable internal causes.

Decreasing performance anxiety

Patients often 'try harder' to fall asleep, but sleep does not respond to being placed under pressure. The patient should be encouraged to try and reduce stress and anxiety levels but not to 'try harder' to fall asleep.

Uncovering faulty beliefs about sleep-promoting practices
Staying in bed longer, reducing social activities, or chasing the mythical 8 hours are not good goals for sleeping better.

Correcting unrealistic sleep expectations
Everyone's sleep requirement is unique, and there is significant intra-individual and night-to-night variability. The patient is taught to be tolerant of their variabilities, and not to compare their sleep needs to the needs of others.

Addressing misattribution of consequences
Patients will experience real daytime consequences of insomnia, but fearing and anticipating them only amplifies the perceived harm. Worry over insomnia can be more problematic than the insomnia itself. Patients are taught to think rationally about the objective consequences of insomnia.

CBT-I

* CBT-I is a multicomponent treatment package, which usually involves three or more insomnia techniques
* Exact components may vary, but usually include:
  * Sleep education
  * Sleep hygiene
  * Stimulus control
  * Sleep restriction
  * Relaxation therapy
  * Cognitive therapy
* Treatment is usually undertaken in four to eight weekly 60–90-minute sessions, though there is evidence supporting briefer courses (i.e. one to two sessions)
* CBT-I can be conducted online, or in person, either individually or in a group (2–15 people) format
* Sleep education and sleep hygiene are not recommended as standalone treatments, but are efficacious within CBT-I models.

Effectiveness of psychological and behavioural interventions

- There is substantial meta-analytic evidence supporting the effectiveness of non-pharmacological interventions for insomnia
- These meta-analyses reveal moderate to large effect sizes for:
  - Reduction in sleep onset latency
  - Reduction in wake after sleep onset
  - Increase in total sleep time
- Studies show that clinical gains are maintained on average for 6–8 months
- The meta-analytic studies included a variety of interventions and the relative efficacy of each component remains unclear
- The AASM states that there is currently insufficient evidence to recommend one single therapy over another or to recommend a single therapy versus multicomponent therapy
- Effect sizes for both brief and group approaches are similar to the effect sizes of individual CBT-I
- A comparison between the objective and subjective effects of CBT-I and common Z drugs on sleep parameters is shown in Table 5.1.

Table 5.1 Comparison of CBT-I, zolpidem, and zopiclone on sleep parameters

Treatment	Decrease in sleep onset latency (min)	Increase in total sleep time (min)	Increase in SE (%)
CBT-I	15.5[a]/33.8[b]	−14.4[a,c]/32.7[b,c]	6.5[a,c]/14.5[b,c]
Zolpidem	6.1[a]/12.8[b]	−51.6[a]/69.2[b]	2.1[a]/2.1[b]
Zopiclone	6.8[a]	−65.6[a]/34.6[b]	−0.8[a]/8.1[b]

[a] Measured by polysomnography. [b] Measured by sleep diary. [c] Average data from two clinical trials comparing CBT-I vs zopiclone and CBT-I vs zolpidem.[1,2] SE, sleep efficiency.

Emerging treatment approaches

There is a vast array of emerging non-pharmacological approaches, none of which currently meet the AASM's standard or recommended threshold.
- Published examples include:
  - Light therapy
  - Mindfulness mediation with CBT-I
  - Acupuncture, acupressure, and electroacupuncture
  - Intensive sleep retraining
  - Biofeedback
- Intensive sleep retraining shows promise for reducing sleep onset latency and increasing total sleep time. The approach is taken over 1 night, where the patient is allowed to sleep for brief periods (up to 3 minutes) before being awakened. The aim is to decondition the insomnia arousal response to sleep onset, thereby resulting in a reduced sleep onset latency
- Biofeedback provides feedback to patients to help them gain control over physiological responses that lead to a decrease in arousal. For example, EMG has been shown to produce similar insomnia improvements to relaxation training. The AASM conclude that the biofeedback can be used with a moderate degree of clinical certainty.

Special populations

Older adults

- Insomnia (especially sleep maintenance) increases across the lifespan for both men and women
- Older age is associated with higher health comorbidities
- Hypnotic use may also be up to five times higher in this group
- Meta-analyses support the use of psychological interventions for insomnia in older adults
- Multicomponent therapy is advised
- A goal of a SE of 85% is strived for instead of the 90% set for younger adults.

Children and teens

- When assessing sleep difficulties in children, developmental stages must be taken into account
- Daytime disturbance is likely to be characterized by irritability, challenging behaviour, and neuropsychological deficits
- CBT-I for children is based on the principles used for adults. However, parents/guardians play a vital role in its implementation
- Techniques specifically used for children include:
  - Extinction treatment
  - Parent training, which is a preventative measure
- Extinction treatment advises that the parent/guardian ignore bedtime tantrums followed by a brief check-in by the parent/guardian
- For more details, see ➜ Chapter 20.

Comorbid insomnia

- The vast majority of insomnia (up to 90%) is comorbid with other mental or physical health conditions
- There is increasing evidence that targeting insomnia in its own right (rather than viewing it as a secondary phenomenon), leads to improvements not only in insomnia but also in comorbid conditions
- The *Diagnostic and Statistical Manual of Mental Disorders*, fifth edition, has replaced primary and secondary insomnia with insomnia disorder to reflect this
- CBT-I has been shown to efficacious in comorbid conditions, including:
  - Chronic pain
  - Fibromyalgia
  - Cancer
  - Alcohol dependence (though it did not influence relapse rates)
  - Depression
  - PTSD (when combined with image rehearsal therapy)
  - Psychosis
  - BPAD (when undertaken by patients who were in-between affective episodes)
- Depending on the comorbidity, the model of CBT-I used may require adaptation, e.g. separately addressing depressed cognitions, which may impact CBT-I concordance in comorbid depression.[3]
- One meta-analysis found a small to medium positive effect size for CBT-I across comorbid conditions, with larger effects for mental health compared to medical comorbidities.[4]

Insomnia and hypnotics

- Medication is often the first-line treatment of insomnia, so it is highly likely that patients presenting for psychological therapy will either have a history of hypnotic use or will currently be taking one
- CBT-I together with hypnotics may have a synergistic effect
- Up to ~85% of patients successfully withdraw from hypnotics using CBT-I, as opposed to ~14% who are told by their clinician to stop
- When to withdraw the hypnotic is very much dependent on each individual patient
- Patients should be advised against suddenly stopping benzodiazepines and the Z drugs (e.g. zopiclone, zolpidem), as there may be a temporary worsening of their insomnia (i.e. rebound insomnia), which can be very distressing. The experience of rebound insomnia may hamper future attempts at withdrawal
- Sleep diaries can be used to help guide withdrawal. In essence, the patient is replacing their hypnotic with CBT-I. An example protocol may include:
  - The patient remains on their hypnotic until a SE of 90% is achieved
  - If possible, the hypnotic dose is then reduced by 25%
  - If the SE remains at 90% the following week, a further dose reduction of 25% can be attempted
  - However, if the SE falls, the patient is advised to remain on their current dose until they regain a SE of 90%. Once they achieve a SE of 90%, further dose reductions are made.

Contraindications

- Patients presenting with the following are usually excluded from CBT-I:
  - Suicidality
  - Terminally ill
  - Excessive alcohol/illicit substance misuse
  - Cognitively impaired (cut off of ≤25 points on the Mini-Mental State Examination)
  - Those undergoing another active psychological therapy
- However, these should not be viewed as absolute contraindications, as depending on the individual there may be scope to work with carers and family members to help implement therapy
- Similarly, CBT-I can be readily incorporated into or complement other therapy types, e.g. a patient undergoing depression-focused psychotherapy could readily incorporate and benefit from CBT-I strategies
- Sleep restriction is contraindicated for patients with bipolar affective disorder, epilepsy, OSA, professional drivers, chronic fatigue syndrome, migraine, or any other condition where sleep loss will exacerbate their comorbid conditions. Sleep compression is advised instead
- Stimulus control is contraindicated for patients with comorbidities: epilepsy, parasomnias, mania, and those at risks of falls
- Sleep restriction and stimulus control are not advised for children and teens.

Risks

- CBT-I is relatively risk-free
- Reduced sleep and increased daytime fatigue are commonly experienced in the early stages of sleep restriction, and patients should be forewarned to expect this (and reassured that it will pass)
- Patients with nocturnal panic are susceptible to the paradoxical phenomenon of relaxation-induced anxiety (up to 15%)
- Sleep restriction, and setting a time in bed of <5 hours for patients with bipolar affective disorder may trigger mania. Sleep compression and a minimum time in bed of 6 hours are advised.

Treatment resistance

- Up to 20% of patients may not respond to CBT-I
- Common reasons for treatment resistance include:
  - A missed comorbid sleep disorder—nocturnal PSG may be helpful here
  - An acute stressful life event
  - Non-concordance
- Patients coming to CBT-I are frequently exhausted and frustrated—they want to sleep better tonight! However, CBT-I takes time to work, and in the early stages, therapy may actually reduce sleep and worsen daytime fatigue
- Throughout CBT-I, it is important to acknowledge and emphasize this. Teaching patients mantras may be helpful as a reinforcer, e.g. 'I am doing this therapy, not to sleep better tonight. In fact, I may sleep worse tonight. I am doing this therapy to sleep better in a few weeks'
- Some patients may be too scared or pessimistic to attempt CBT-I. The process of creative hopelessness may help patients to recognize that their current approach is not working or sustainable. Patients can probably cite a long list of the failed strategies they've employed. Ask 'As a result of all these efforts, has your sleep gotten better or worse?' and 'Has your quality of life gotten better or worse?' They already know the results if they continue to do what they are doing. Might they be willing to try something different?

Relapse prevention

- Insomnia is often a persistent and relapsing–remitting condition
- It takes time for a patient to build confidence in the psychological and behavioural techniques they have learned. In the initial recovery period, patients will often fear relapse
- Addressing this fear at the end of therapy is helpful, as well as advising further sources of support, e.g. bibliotherapy (see 'Further reading')
- In the face of relapse, a patient could be advised to:
  - *Detect*: recommence sleep diaries and sleep *restriction*
  - *Detach*: reinstate stimulus control
  - *Distract*: recommence cognitive and relaxation techniques.

Further reading

Guidelines

American Academy of Sleep Medicine. Psychological and pharmacological treatment of insomnia—practice guidelines. Available at:https://aasm.org/clinical-resources/practice-standards/practice-guidelines/

National Institute for Health and Care Excellence. Insomnia. 2021. Available at: 🔗 https://cks.nice.org.uk/insomnia

For patients

Espie CA. Overcoming Insomnia and Sleep Problems: A Self-Help Guide Using Cognitive Behavioral Techniques. London: Robinson; 2006.

Anderson KA. How to Beat Insomnia and Sleep Problems One Step at a Time: Using evidence-based low-intensity CBT; 2018.

For clinicians

Perlis ML. Cognitive Behavioral Treatment of Insomnia: A Session-by-Session Guide. New York: Springer; 2008.

Perlis ML, Aloia M, Kuhn BR. Behavioral treatments for sleep disorders: A Comprehensive Primer of Behavioral Sleep Medicine Interventions. Amsterdam: Academic; 2011.

References

1. Sivertsen B, Omvik S, Pallesen S, et al. Cognitive behavioral therapy vs. zopiclone for treatment of chronic primary insomnia in older adults. JAMA. 2006;295(24):2851–8.
2. Mitchell MD, Gehrman P, Perlis M et al. Comparative effectiveness of cognitive behavioral therapy for insomnia: a systematic review. BMC Fam Pract. 2012;13:40.
3. O'Regan D. Cognitive behaviour therapy for insomnia in co-morbid psychiatric disorder. In: Selsick H (Ed) Sleep Disorders in Psychiatric Patients A Practical Guide. Berlin: Springer; 2018:149–74.
4. Wu JQ, Appleman ER, Salazar RD, et al. Cognitive behavioral therapy for insomnia comorbid with psychiatric and medical conditions: a meta-analysis. JAMA Intern Med. 2015;175(9):1461–72.

Medical management of insomnia

Hugh Selsick

Introduction

Treatment of insomnia often requires medication. The range of licensed hypnotics differ from country to country but there are generally only a few drugs specifically licensed for insomnia. As a result, it is not uncommon for unlicensed medications to be used as well. The evidence base for the long-term use of hypnotics and the use of unlicensed medications in insomnia is scant, but clinical experience and an understanding of the underlying pharmacology can fill in some of the gaps in the scientific literature.

Neurotransmitters in insomnia treatment

In order to fully understand the medical management of insomnia, it is helpful to appreciate the role of certain important neurotransmitters and hormones which impact sleep–wake regulation. These can be divided into two categories (Table 6.1):

- Neurotransmitters that promote wakefulness. Drugs which counteract these neurotransmitters can promote sleep
- Neurotransmitters/hormones that promote sleep. Drugs which enhance or mimic the activity of these neurotransmitters promote sleep.

Table 6.1 Neurotransmitters and hormones involved in sleep–wake regulation

Promote wakefulness	Promote sleep
Noradrenaline	GABA
Serotonin	Melatonin
Acetylcholine	Adenosine[b]
Histamine	
Glutamate	
Orexin/hypocretin	
Dopamine[a]	

[a] Raising dopamine levels promotes wakefulness, but its role in the unmedicated brain is less certain.

[b] There are no adenosine promoting drugs and so this neurotransmitter will not be discussed further.

Mode of action of licensed hypnotics

Licensed hypnotics primarily act through the following mechanisms:
- Positive allosteric modulators of $GABA_A$ (i.e. enhance GABA function), e.g. benzodiazepines, zopiclone, and zolpidem
- Melatonin and melatonin agonists, e.g. ramelteon (not available in the UK), melatonin modified release
- Histamine antagonists, e.g. promethazine
- Orexin antagonists, e.g. suvorexant (not available in the UK)
- Chloral hydrate (mechanism of action unknown) and clomethiazole (GABA mimetic) are rarely used in clinical practice and are not discussed further.

Drugs that act on GABA~A~ receptors

Drugs that act on GABA$_A$ receptors

These comprise the vast majority of hypnotics and are broadly divided into the benzodiazepines and the so-called Z drugs. They enhance GABA's sedative activity to promote sleep. The drugs in this class differ in their receptor specificity and their pharmacokinetics.

Table 6.2 outlines the pharmacokinetic properties of the GABA type A (GABA$_A$) receptor positive allosteric modulators.[1-4] It is important to note that these figures are subject to significant variability as some drugs have active metabolites and their pharmacokinetics will be affected by age, liver and kidney disease, and the presence of other interacting drugs.

Table 6.2 Pharmacokinetics of commonly used benzodiapines and Z drugs

Drug	Absorption	Half-life (hours)	Active metabolite half-life (hours)
Diazepam	Rapid	20–100	30–90
Flurazepam	Rapid	2	30–100
Loprazolam	Slow	8	7
Lormetazepam	Rapid	13	–
Nitrazepam	Intermediate	24	30–90
Oxazepam	Rapid	7	–
Temazepam	Slow	10	–
Zaleplon	Rapid	1	–
Zolpidem	Rapid	2	–
Zopiclone	Rapid	4	3–6

For these drugs, the degree of sedation is generally correlated with the plasma level. Understanding the differences in pharmacokinetics can therefore help with selecting the best drug for your patient:
- Rapidly absorbed drugs are useful for initial insomnia
- More slowly absorbed drugs may be useful for middle-of-the-night insomnia. They should be taken at bedtime so that their peak sedative effect coincides with the period of wakefulness in the night
- If the patient only has initial insomnia, with no difficulty maintaining sleep, shorter half-life drugs are a good choice
- If they have difficulty with sleep maintenance, or both sleep initiation and sleep maintenance, then a longer half-life drug may be better
- Longer half-life drugs have the potential to cause daytime sedation and should be avoided if this sedation is undesirable
- In patients who take the drug on a nightly basis, there is the risk of accumulation with longer half-life drugs. In these patients, shorter-acting drugs are preferred. If patients only use the medication intermittently, this is less of an issue
- Older adults and patients with kidney or liver dysfunction are also at risk of drug accumulation and thus shorter-acting drugs may be safer.

Melatonin and melatonin agonists

Melatonin, as a 2 mg modified-release tablet, is a prescription-only drug in the UK and some other countries, but in many countries it is not classed as a medication and is available off the shelf. There have not been many long-term studies of safety and efficacy, but the existing studies, and the lack of reports of any serious adverse events despite its wide availability is reassuring.[5]

- Ramelteon is a melatonin agonist licensed for insomnia treatment in the US where it is licensed for long-term use. It is not available in the UK
- Melatonin modified release (Circadin®) is licensed for 13 weeks in over 55s
- However, it is widely used off licence in younger adults and children
- In research studies and clinical practice, both significantly lower and higher doses are frequently used. There is no widely agreed dose range for melatonin
- Melatonin has a half-life of 45 minutes and Circadin® has a half-life of 3.5–4 hours.[6] As a result, morning sedation is usually not a problem.

Antihistamines

- Over-the-counter antihistamines are widely used as hypnotics despite a paucity of good evidence for their efficacy and safety, particularly with long-term use
- Sedating antihistamines also tend to have significant anticholinergic activity which leads to sedation, constipation, dry mouth, and other short-term side effects. In longer-term use, anticholinergic drugs may raise the risk of dementia
- Many sedating antidepressants and antipsychotics also have antihistamine activity which contributes to their sedative properties. Some of these have anticholinergic properties as well, but often not to the same extent as antihistamines
- Antihistaminergic drugs are generally long acting and may produce their peak sedative effects some time after the peak plasma level.[7] They can therefore be useful in the treatment of middle-of-the-night insomnia or early morning waking.

Antidepressants

It is a common misperception that all antidepressants are sedative. Indeed, most of the newer antidepressants such as the selective serotonin reuptake inhibitors and the serotonin and noradrenaline reuptake inhibitors are more likely to be activating and may exacerbate insomnia. There are, however, a number of sedating antidepressants that are widely used (often at doses below the antidepressant threshold) to treat insomnia. On the other hand, where there is comorbid insomnia and depression/anxiety, there is a strong case for using a sedative antidepressant at antidepressant doses to treat both conditions with a single drug.

- Amitriptyline is widely used to treat insomnia in clinical practice. There is some evidence that it may be effective, but it can lead to significant daytime sedation and the anticholinergic side effects limit its use as a first-line drug
- Trazodone is useful in insomnia and can be combined with activating antidepressants to counteract the sleep disruption caused by these medications. It may be a good choice in insomnia in the context of post-traumatic stress disorder as it reduces nightmares
- Mirtazapine is often effective in treating insomnia and can also be used to counteract the sleep disruptive effects of activating antidepressants. Increased hunger with weight gain is problematic for some patients.[8]

Practical considerations when prescribing for insomnia

When should you prescribe hypnotics?

Hypnotics should be considered when:

- Insomnia is likely to short lived. For example, hypnotics can be useful if there is a clear stressor that is likely to resolve in the near future, or when starting on an antidepressant such as a selective serotonin reuptake inhibitor, which may cause a transient worsening of insomnia
- Insomnia is chronic and causing significant distress. Cognitive behavioural therapy should always be considered as a first line in the management of chronic insomnia, but hypnotics may have a role while the patient is waiting for therapy
- Insomnia is adversely affecting the patient's mental health
- The patient has not responded to cognitive behaviour therapy or the therapy is not available
- Substance misuse where the substance is clearly being used to self-medicate for insomnia. It may be safer to prescribe a hypnotic than for the patient to drink to excess or self-medicate with sedatives. In this case, it is essential to check that the patient has stopped using the substance once they have started the hypnotic
- Insomnia is sporadic and the medication is likely to be used only occasionally.

When do you want the drug to work?

Your choice of medication will largely be determined by what time of night the insomnia occurs.

Difficulty falling asleep:

- If the problem is purely one of sleep initiation, it is best to use short-acting medications with a quick onset of action. This ensures the patient doesn't need to take the medication too far in advance of bedtime and is less likely to experience morning hangover
- Zolpidem and melatonin are sensible choices
- If there is difficulty in both initiating and maintaining sleep, then a longer-acting drug such as zopiclone or temazepam may be better.

Difficulty staying asleep:

- Longer-acting drugs taken at bedtime are the only option currently available
- Zopiclone or temazepam may be useful though early morning waking can still be a problem
- Antihistaminergic drugs are often used with good effect.

How important is it to avoid morning hangover?

There are certain patients where avoiding morning hangover is highly desirable:

- Elderly patients: morning sedation may raise the risk of falls
- Drivers: longer-acting hypnotics can impair driving performance
- Safety critical profession: where any reduction in attention may be hazardous.

In these patients, a shorter-acting hypnotic such as melatonin or zolpidem is preferred. However, it is important to note that there is a great deal of variability between patients in terms of how sedated they may feel after taking a particular drug and patients may not always be good judges of how much their alertness is impaired.

Comorbid conditions

The presence of comorbid conditions may dictate the choice of medication. Other medical and psychiatric disorders may preclude the use of certain drugs and interactions between the hypnotics and the other medications need to be considered. However, comorbid conditions can also help with the choice of appropriate medications. Where possible, one should avoid polypharmacy and therefore, if possible, select a drug that treats both the insomnia and the comorbid condition:

- Sedative antidepressants can be taken at night to improve both depression and insomnia
- Amitriptyline, when used for pain, may improve insomnia symptoms
- Patients with insomnia who require antipsychotics for psychosis or as mood stabilizers could be prescribed more sedating antipsychotics. These should be loaded at night as far as possible
- Allergy sufferers can be treated with sedating antihistamines at night if insomnia is a problem.

Other factors to consider include:

- In psychiatric patients at higher risk of suicide, the hypnotics should be prescribed in smaller quantities to minimize the risk of overdose
- Hypnotics, when used in licensed doses, do not appear to worsen OSA and so untreated sleep apnoea is not necessarily a contraindication to their use[9]
- Start with lower doses and titrate more slowly in patients with liver or kidney disease.

Addiction

Addiction is a potential problem with hypnotics, but it is not inevitable. Indeed, most patients who use hypnotics, even those who use them frequently, do not become addicted. Long-term use of a hypnotic does not necessarily mean the patient is addicted to it; insomnia is often a long-term condition and therefore may require long-term medication. However, the risk of addiction should be discussed with patients and carers and these risks should be weighed up against the risk of having untreated insomnia.

Stopping hypnotics

There are a number of circumstances where one may decide to stop a hypnotic:

- The insomnia has resolved or the stressor driving the insomnia has been removed
- The patient has started an alternative treatment such as cognitive behaviour therapy for insomnia or a sedating antidepressant
- The patient has unacceptable side effects
- The patient is abusing the drug, e.g. using it above the licensed dose or using it in the day.

There are no hard and fast rules about how to stop long-term hypnotics but the following guidelines are helpful:

- Prescribe the drug in the smallest possible denomination tablet to allow for a gradual decrease in dose
- Reduce the dose by 25% every 1–2 weeks
- Set target dates for each reduction but be flexible
- Warn the patients that they may experience a temporary worsening of their insomnia (rebound insomnia) and that this will resolve with time
- Monitor their progress closely and adjust the rate of reduction where needed. A patient can still take a full dose of the medication on occasional nights even if they are reducing their dose on other nights
- Similarly, once a patient is no longer taking the drug regularly, they may still need it on occasional nights.

References

1. Anderson IM, McAllister-Williams RH. Fundamentals of Clinical Psychopharmacology. 4th ed. Boca Raton, FL: CRC Press; 2016.
2. Breimer DD. Pharmacokinetics and metabolism of various benzodiazepines used as hypnotics. Br J Clin Pharmacol. 1979;8(1):7S–13S.
3. Clark BG, Jue SG, Dawson GW, et al. Loprazolam. A preliminary review of its pharmacodynamic and pharmacokinetic properties and therapeutic efficacy in insomnia. Drugs. 1986;31(6):500–16.
4. Hümpel M, Illi V, Milius W, et al. The pharmacokinetics and biotransformation of the new benzodiazepine lormetazepam in humans. I. Absorption, distribution, elimination and metabolism of lormetazepam-5-14C. Eur J Drug Metab Pharmacokinet. 1979;4(4):237–43.
5. Andersen LP, Gögenur I, Rosenberg J, et al. The safety of melatonin in humans. Clin Drug Investig. 2016;36(3):169–75.
6. Harpsøe NG, Andersen LP, Gögenur I, et al. Clinical pharmacokinetics of melatonin: a systematic review. Eur J Clin Pharmacol. 2015;71(8):901–909.
7. Krystal AD, Richelson E, Roth T. Review of the histamine system and the clinical effects of H1 antagonists: basis for a new model for understanding the effects of insomnia medications. Sleep Med Rev. 2013;17(4):263–72.
8. Aszalós Z. Effects of antidepressants on sleep. Orvosi Hetilap. 2006;147(17):773–83.
9. Mason M, Cates CJ, Smith I. Effects of opioid, hypnotic and sedating medications on sleep-disordered breathing in adults with obstructive sleep apnoea. Cochrane Database Syst Rev. 2015;7:CD011090.

Sleep-disordered breathing

Joerg Steier and *Brian Kent*

Introduction

Respiratory function is significantly altered by sleep. People with entirely normal breathing when awake can develop very significant respiratory compromise during sleep. Following sleep onset, central motor neuron output falls. This means that diminished upper airway dilator muscle function leads to a narrower upper airway, while reduced inspiratory muscle activity causes a shallower breathing pattern compared to the awake state.

Changes in respiratory physiology with sleep onset include:
- Reduced central motor neuron output
- Narrowed upper airway, potentially causing snoring or obstruction
- Reduced inspiratory muscle activity and lower respiratory rate, contributing to a shallower breathing pattern
- Reduced chemoreceptor sensitivity
- Reduced minute ventilation.

These physiological changes occur in everyone, but may become problematic if combined with one or more complicating factors:
- Obesity
- Enlarged neck circumference
- Obstruction of the upper airway, e.g. enlarged tonsils, adenoids, or polyps
- Kinking of the airway
- Retrognathia
- Chronic obstructive or restrictive ventilatory defects.

Any abnormal breathing at night leading to symptoms, sleep disturbance, or long-term complications is labelled sleep-disordered breathing (SDB).

Classification

Depending on the pathophysiology and severity, there are different types of SDB:
- Snoring
- Upper airway resistance syndrome (UARS)
- Obstructive sleep apnoea (OSA)
- Central sleep apnoea (CSA)
- Complex sleep apnoea
- Obesity hypoventilation syndrome (OHS)
- Hypercapnic respiratory failure associated with chronic obstructive pulmonary disease
- Hypoventilation syndromes due to other neuromuscular conditions
- Rare conditions, e.g. Ondine's curse.

Epidemiology

Snoring is common and affects up to half of middle-aged male subjects. It becomes more common with obesity or following exposure to centrally inhibiting agents, such as alcohol or sedatives.

If the upper airway obstruction causes high inspiratory work of breathing, then this leads to UARS. Once the upper airway collapses entirely this is called OSA.

- OSA is the most common type of SDB
- Current estimates suggest that anywhere up to 23% of middle-aged women and 49% of middle-aged men may have at least moderate levels of OSA
- With the obesity epidemic, rates of OSA have risen worldwide.

Other forms of SDB are less common. OHS is increasing in prevalence as the global population becomes more obese, with a prevalence of ~0.4% in the general population.

Definition

SDB can affect sleep quality and quantity in different ways:
- Sleep fragmentation
- Intermittent hypoxia
- Intrathoracic pressure swings
- Hypercapnia.

The severity of SDB is typically defined by the frequency of respiratory events. The AHI counts the numbers of respiratory events and divides it by the sleep time (in hours). The respiratory disturbance index (RDI) also includes the number of respiratory arousals caused by respiratory effort and is used to diagnose UARS. See Fig. 7.1.

The AHI and the RDI have the following thresholds:
- 0–5 events/hour indicates normal breathing
- 5–15 events/hour indicates mild SDB
- 15–30 events/hour indicates moderate SDB
- >30 events/hour indicates severe SDB.

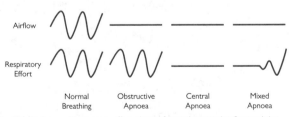

Fig. 7.1 Airflow and inspiratory effort plotted for unobstructed airflow and the different types of apnoeas.

Clinical features

Patients with SDB may present with a wide variety of nocturnal and daytime symptoms:

- Snoring
- Observed apnoeas or hypopnoeas
- Restless and broken sleep
- Waking with choking or gasping
- Nocturia
- Nocturnal gastric reflux
- Dry mouth, particularly in the mornings
- Morning headaches
- Daytime sleepiness
- Memory problems, diminished concentration
- Mood abnormalities like depression
- Other physiological dysfunction, such as treatment-resistant hypertension, libido problems, and so on.

In patients with sleep disorders, the bed partner's observations are an essential part of the clinical history. Screening for SDB using questionnaires (e.g. Epworth Sleepiness Scale, STOP-Bang questionnaire) and sleep studies is still contentious, but may be most useful in at-risk populations such as bariatric patients.

Obstructive sleep apnoea

Obstructive sleep apnoea is characterized by upper airway obstruction during sleep, but with maintained breathing effort (➔ Fig. 7.1, p. 71). OSA is the most common type of SDB of medical concern. In recent decades, OSA prevalence has increased in line with obesity rates, and nowadays it is thought that it might affect up to 10% of middle-aged male and 3% of middle-aged female subjects.

Degrees of severity:
• Mild OSA: AHI 5–15/hour
• Moderate OSA: AHI 15–30/hour
• Severe OSA: AHI >30/hour.

Apnoeas and hypopnoeas trigger oxygen desaturations, and the oxygen desaturation index (ODI) recorded by nocturnal pulse oximetry can be used as a surrogate marker for the AHI. When OSA occurs in combination with excessive daytime sleepiness, the condition is labelled as OSA syndrome. However, there is little correlation between symptoms and AHI severity.

OSA is strongly associated with, and may worsen, the following conditions (➔ Chapters 8 and 23):
• Cardiovascular disease, and in particular hypertension
• Type 2 diabetes
• Cognitive impairment
• Mood disorders
• Respiratory diseases, such as asthma and interstitial lung disease
• Gastro-oesophageal reflux disease.

Generic therapeutic recommendations may include:
• Weight loss, if indicated
• Avoidance of sleeping in a supine posture
• Avoidance of sedatives, centrally relaxing agents, and alcohol.

In addition to these, specific therapy may be indicated to control upper airway patency while asleep:
• Continuous positive airway pressure (CPAP), (➔ Chapter 9)
• Mandibular advancement device (➔ Chapter 10)
• Ear, nose, and throat (ENT) review to optimize upper airway patency, e.g. to excise enlarged tonsils, polyps, and adenoids (➔ Chapter 11)
• Other special therapies may be required, e.g. non-invasive ventilation, surgery, or novel therapies (➔ Chapter 12).

Upper airway resistance syndrome

When falling asleep, the neuromuscular tone to the dilator muscles of the airway falls and the upper airway narrows. If this leads to a significant rise in resistance to airflow, then inspiratory effort might increase until the patient wakes with an arousal from sleep, but without the apnoeas, hypopnoeas, or desaturations of OSA. This fragments sleep and can leave the patient excessively sleepy.

In UARS, patients continue to breathe and do not desaturate. The AHI and ODI are therefore insufficient tools to characterize UARS. To identify respiratory arousals caused by respiratory effort, the RDI evaluates EEG arousals, and as a result PSG is needed to make a formal diagnosis of UARS. The treatment of UARS is similar to that of OSA (◗ Obstructive sleep apnoea, p. 73).

Central sleep apnoea

CSA differs from OSA in that there is no central inspiratory effort, and the upper airway does not necessarily collapse. CSA is commonly associated with the following conditions:

- Heart failure (>50% of patients with New York Heart Association class III–IV heart failure have CSA)
- Acute or chronic neurological conditions affecting brainstem function (e.g. stroke, posterior fossa space-occupying lesion)
- Medication use:
  - Opiates
  - Sedatives (e.g. benzodiazepines)
  - Gabapentinoids
- Alcohol consumption
- Altitude.

CSA is of particular clinical relevance in heart failure. A subtype of CSA, Cheyne–Stokes respiration, is characterized by a crescendo–decrescendo pattern, wherein periods of vigorous respiratory effort will gradually dwindle away until breathing temporarily ceases. CSA/Cheyne–Stokes respiration is typically seen in patients with suboptimally controlled, severe heart failure, and predicts an increased risk of negative outcomes.

While CPAP therapy can be used for the treatment of CSA, there is little evidence that it improves any long-term outcomes. A related treatment to control CSA is adaptive servo-ventilation, where pressure and flow are altered in response to changes in breathing. Adaptive servo-ventilation effectively abolishes CSA, but does not reduce—and may worsen—mortality outcomes in patients with significant heart failure.

Consequently, the treatment of CSA usually involves attempts to improve or remove the underlying causal factors, whether related to heart failure or medication use.

Patients who develop CSA when they are treated for OSA with CPAP have what is termed 'complex sleep apnoea'. Complex sleep apnoea occurs because long-standing OSA has caused ventilatory instability, with markedly altered sensitivity to CO_2 levels leading to recurrent episodes of CSA while on CPAP. Complex sleep apnoea will usually resolve without specific intervention, but may occasionally require treatment with adaptive servo-ventilation or other more advanced forms of positive airway pressure (PAP) therapy.

Hypoventilation

Nocturnal hypoventilation is caused by an insufficient minute ventilation (reduced breathing with consequent reduced gas exchange) when asleep. It causes nocturnal prolonged oxygen desaturations and raised levels of CO_2, and can contribute to acute and chronic respiratory failure, putting patients at risk. Patients with hypoventilation are at increased risk of pulmonary hypertension and consequent heart failure.

Hypoventilation is typically caused by one of the following:
- Increased load on the respiratory muscle pump (e.g. in OHS) or with increased airway resistance (chronic obstructive pulmonary disease)
- Diminished capacity of the respiratory muscle pump (e.g. in myopathies, dystrophies, myasthenia gravis, spinal cord injury/trauma, stroke)
- Inability to sustain sufficient neural respiratory drive when asleep (e.g. Ondine's curse, stroke).

Certain modifying factors may influence the occurrence of nocturnal periods of hypoventilation:
- Posture: in supine sleep, the intra-abdominal pressures splint the diaphragm and impose a threshold load on the inspiratory muscles; lateral or prone posture are generally favourable to diminish the impact of SDB
- Sleep stage: during REM sleep, physiological atonia of the skeletal muscles—other than the diaphragm and the external eye muscles—develops, and patients who depend on accessory muscle activity to maintain adequate respiratory effort may then develop significant periods of hypoventilation.

Treatment of hypoventilation often requires extrinsic support of the respiratory muscle pump, as it is caused by 'pump failure'. Consequently, mere splinting of the upper airway with CPAP therapy may not be sufficient, and formal non-invasive ventilation with a bi-level pressure support mode may be required to provide adequate nocturnal ventilation.

When the problem causing nocturnal hypoventilation continues into wakefulness, then patients develop daytime hypercapnic respiratory failure. Measuring venous bicarbonate appears to be a useful screening tool for evolving hypoventilation; elevations in serum bicarbonate are seen before significant changes in daytime partial pressure of oxygen (PO_2) and partial pressure of CO_2 (PCO_2) levels.

Comorbidities of sleep-disordered breathing

SDB has an intimate relationship with a number of comorbid factors. Some of these may cause or worsen SDB, while SDB may contribute to the development or progression of others:

- Obesity—increased body mass contributes to the development of snoring, OSA, and OHS
- Neurological conditions or heart failure causing CSA
- Metabolic abnormalities that cause acidosis or alkalosis, and compensatory mechanisms leading to hyper- or hypoventilation with apnoeas
- Use of certain types of drugs, e.g. alcohol, opiates, and sedatives, typically causing hypoventilation and CSA
- SDB increases sympathetic drive which has negative effects on blood pressure and heart failure (➜ Chapter 8)
- SDB is associated with a higher risk of diabetes, and with worse diabetic control (➜ Chapter 8)
- During pregnancy, OSA can be caused by increased amounts of body fluid that narrow the upper airway during sleep. This may be associated with an increased risk of pre-eclampsia and adverse perinatal outcomes.

Further reading

Hosselet J, Ayappa I, Norman RG, et al. Classification of sleep-disordered breathing. Am J Respir Crit Care Med. 2001;163(2):398–405.
Muza RT. Central sleep apnoea—a clinical review. J Thorac Dis. 2015;7(5):930–37.
Veasey SC, Rosen IM. Obstructive sleep apnea in adults. N Engl J Med. 2019;380(15):1442–49.

Sleep-disordered breathing and its associations

Brian Kent

Introduction

People with OSA can be affected by a huge variety of unpleasant symptoms, ranging from broken nocturnal sleep and nocturia, to overwhelming daytime sleepiness and low mood. They also are more likely to be involved in car crashes, and to have significantly impaired concentration and daytime functioning. However, a combination of sleepiness, cognitive or psychological symptoms, and an incremental reduction in overall economic productivity are unlikely to cause undue public or scientific excitement. Where OSA becomes more relevant from a population health perspective is in its relationship with long-term illness and death, a relationship largely mediated through an apparent effect of OSA on the likelihood of people developing cardiovascular and metabolic disease, and possibly also cancer. Longitudinal observational studies consistently show that increasing OSA severity is associated with excess morbidity and mortality, above and beyond the expected effects of confounding factors such as obesity.

Obstructive sleep apnoea and cardiovascular disease

Mechanisms of cardiovascular disease in OSA

Patients with OSA experience sleep fragmentation and intermittent hypoxia. Each of these appears capable of increasing cardiovascular risk, but recent data would suggest that intermittent hypoxia may be the more important of the two. This risk seems to be mediated via a number of pathophysiological mechanisms:

* Sympathetic overactivity, substantially due to central and peripheral chemoreceptor stimulation by transient hypoxaemia and hypercapnia
* Chronic systemic inflammation
* Oxidative stress, due to the generation of reactive oxygen species
* Metabolic dysfunction.

These factors combine to cause endothelial dysfunction, increased arterial stiffness, and subsequently atherosclerosis and clinically overt cardiovascular disease.

Additionally, a number of local and mechanical factors due to regional hypoxia and attempts to inspire against an obstructed upper airway may predispose to the development of systemic and pulmonary hypertension:

* Increased right ventricular pre-load due to negative intrathoracic pressure
* Hypoxic pulmonary artery vasoconstriction leading to increased right ventricular afterload
* Impaired left ventricular filling due to right ventricular distension and septal displacement
* Increased left ventricular afterload due to increased left ventricular transmural pressure.

These mechanical effects may be of particular relevance in patients with heart failure and concomitant OSA.

Cardiovascular outcomes in OSA patients

A diagnosis of moderate to severe OSA appears to confer an increased risk of cardiovascular disease:

* Hypertension risk is increased approximately threefold
* Symptomatic coronary artery disease risk is increased approximately fourfold in sleep clinic populations with severe OSA, and by ~70% in community-based populations of middle-aged men with severe OSA
* Stroke risk increases by ~300% in men with severe OSA, but this relationship is not seen in women
* Heart failure in ~60% more likely to develop in men with severe OSA; again, this relationship is much weaker in women
* Atrial fibrillation is approximately twice as likely to occur in subjects with OSA.

A diagnosis of OSA is also associated with increased mortality in patients with established coronary artery disease or heart failure, and may lead to worse functional outcomes in stroke patients.

On the other hand, it is also possible that OSA may have a slightly counterintuitive protective effect in some people. This is postulated to be due to the phenomenon of ischaemic preconditioning, whereby myocardium and brain tissue are made better equipped to deal with periods of ischaemia by recurrent episodes of transient hypoxia leading to the development of local adaptive mechanisms. This may particularly be the case in people with milder OSA, or older OSA patients. Conclusive data to support this hypothesis do not as yet exist, however.

Treatment of OSA and cardiovascular outcomes

Treating OSA with CPAP has a robust and consistent effect on hypertension in randomized controlled trials:

- CPAP therapy seems to cause a reduction of systolic blood pressure of about 3 mmHg. This is of questionable importance at an individual level, but may be of relevance at a population level
- CPAP used alone is not a highly effective antihypertensive; studies comparing it with antihypertensive drugs such as valsartan suggest that medication has a much greater effect on blood pressure reduction
- OSA is particularly common in patients with resistant hypertension, where CPAP may be a useful adjunctive therapy.

Retrospective studies have suggested that treating OSA may have a very meaningful effect on long-term cardiovascular risk. In a large Spanish sleep clinic population, untreated severe OSA was associated with a threefold likelihood of cardiac death over 12 years of follow-up, an association that was not observed in patients who received CPAP. Retrospective studies are of course vulnerable to a host of biases, and recent prospective randomized controlled trials have not found that CPAP therapy reduces medium-term cardiac risk in patients with established cardiovascular disease. A number of caveats somewhat limit the generalizability of the findings of these randomized controlled trials, however:

- They excluded patients who were sleepy
- They included patients with fairly modest levels of OSA
- They examined the utility of CPAP in secondary prevention, rather than primary prevention, of cardiac morbidity
- Adherence to CPAP therapy in these studies is rather poor, generally averaging around 3 hours per night.

In summary, OSA has multiple physiological consequences that should increase cardiovascular risk, and people with OSA indeed appear to be at increased risk of developing cardiovascular disease. It is not clear at this point, however, if treating OSA leads to improved cardiovascular outcomes, beyond a relatively modest reduction in blood pressure.

OSA and metabolic disease

As mentioned previously, one of the ways in which OSA may exert a negative influence on long-term cardiovascular health is through its relationship with metabolic disease. OSA has a particularly intimate relationship with insulin resistance and type 2 diabetes mellitus (T2D):

- OSA is found in between 15% and 30% of people with T2D
- Between 23% and 86% of diabetics have OSA

- Following adjustment for obesity and other confounding factors, patients with severe OSA are twice as likely to have T2D or pre-diabetes than non-apnoeic people
- A diagnosis of severe OSA increases the risk of subsequently developing T2D by about 30%
- Diabetic OSA patients are twice as likely to have poorly controlled T2D
- Diabetic OSA patients are more likely to develop retinopathy.

The mechanisms underlying any association between OSA and T2D are rather similar to those mentioned earlier regarding cardiovascular disease. White adipose tissue may be particularly important here—in obese people, white adipose tissue functions as a significant endocrine organ mediating glucose metabolism. Sympathetic overactivity and local tissue hypoxia cause white adipose tissue to become inflamed and resistant to insulin signalling, with intermittent hypoxia potentially having a particularly negative effect. OSA may also have a deleterious effect on hepatic glucose metabolism and may also contribute to pancreatic B-cell dysfunction.

Does treating OSA lead to better diabetic control?

The short answer is, we're not sure:

- Uncontrolled studies generally show that successful treatment of OSA is associated with reduced insulin resistance and reduced glycated haemoglobin (HbA1c) levels
- Rigid adherence to CPAP therapy for 2 weeks in patients admitted to a sleep laboratory leads to reduced insulin resistance
- The short-term withdrawal of CPAP therapy in patients with established OSA leads to increased nocturnal glucose levels
- Randomized controlled trials have produced conflicting results regarding the effect of CPAP therapy on HbA1c levels, but the largest study to date found no effect
- The only randomized controlled trial examining the impact of treating OSA on complications of T2D found no benefit from 12 months of CPAP therapy on eyesight.

An intriguing potential explanation for the apparent futility of trying to treat T2D (or for that matter, cardiovascular disease) with CPAP is the apparent differential impact on HbA1c of OSA occurring during REM versus NREM sleep. REM-OSA appears to have a much stronger relationship with HbA1c levels than OSA occurring during NREM sleep, and if a high proportion of diabetics given CPAP for their OSA choose to stop treatment halfway through the night, the vast bulk of their REM-OSA will remain untreated.

As with cardiovascular disease, although fairly robust evidence supports a causal link between OSA and T2D, the utility of CPAP as an antidiabetic agent remains weak at present.

OSA and cancer

Perhaps a little surprisingly, a diagnosis of OSA may increase the risk of developing, and of dying from, cancer. Longitudinal observational studies from Europe, North America, and Australia have found that more severe OSA—and in particular, more severe nocturnal hypoxaemia—is associated with a roughly twofold risk of incident cancer, and up to a fivefold risk of cancer mortality. While the findings of some other studies suggest that any increase in cancer risk in patients with OSA might simply be due to established carcinogenic factors such as smoking and obesity, an increasing body of evidence from *in vitro* and animal studies supports the notion that OSA may by itself promote oncogenesis.

Potential causative mechanisms include intermittent hypoxia-related systemic inflammation and oxidative stress, tumour hypoxia leading to increased cell proliferation and angiogenesis, and OSA-related alterations in antitumour immune function.

Future studies will try and tease out which types of cancer are most likely to be influenced by OSA (at the moment, the strongest link is probably with melanoma), and the effect of treating OSA on cancer outcomes.

OSA and neurodegenerative disease

It is clear that untreated OSA will lead to impairment of daytime functioning in a significant proportion of people with the disease, but emerging evidence suggests that it may also increase the risk of subsequent cognitive impairment, and in particular of Alzheimer's disease (AD). Indeed, patients with appear to be about five times more likely than matched controls to have coexistent OSA.

Putative contributory factors to an increased risk of AD and cognitive impairment in OSA patients are (as before) postulated to largely be attributable to sleep fragmentation and intermittent hypoxia, and include:

- Neuroinflammation
- Alterations in permeability of the blood–brain barrier
- Reduced clearance of beta-amyloid by the glymphatic system
- Cerebrovascular disease.

The study of the relationship between OSA and AD remains in its (relative) infancy, and confirmatory longitudinal studies are needed. More to the point, although treating OSA in early AD might seem an attractive potentially disease-modifying option, experience with other diseases seemingly caused or worsened by OSA tells us that treating SDB doesn't always lead to the expected improvements in comorbidities.

For more details, see ➜ Chapter 23.

Conclusion

A significant body of evidence suggests that OSA contributes to the development and progression of a number of important comorbid diseases. Unfortunately, current treatment modalities for OSA seem to have a relatively limited impact on these diseases.

Further reading

Almendros I, Gozal D. Intermittent hypoxia and cancer: undesirable bed partners? Respir Physiol Neurobiol. 2018;256:79–86.

Mandal S, Kent BD. Obstructive sleep apnoea and coronary artery disease. J Thorac Dis. 2018;10(Suppl 34):S4212–20.

Reutrakul S, Mokhlesi B. Obstructive sleep apnea and diabetes: a state of the art review. Chest. 2017;152(5):1070–86.

Rosenzweig I, Glasser M, Polsek D, et al. Sleep apnoea and the brain: a complex relationship. Lancet Respir Med. 2015;3(5):404–14.

Medical management of sleep-disordered breathing

Adrian J. Williams

Introduction

Strategies addressing the underdiagnosis of OSA, which is a barrier to effective treatment, are important, e.g.:

- Increasing patient awareness of the symptoms
- Validated questionnaires, such as the STOP-Bang questionnaire, used effectively in mandatory preoperative assessments
- Physician awareness of the symptoms of snoring, witnessed apnoeas and sleepiness, especially in the overweight, and referral for respiratory sleep studies.

Elimination of contributing factors, such as:

- Obesity (with a 10% reduction in weight, there is a 25% reduction in apnoeas and hypopneas). Advice revolves around reduced food intake and increased energy expenditure
- Nasal obstruction-an increase in resistance to nasal breathing is associated with an increase in negative intrathoracic pressure which is transmitted to the pharyngeal airway promoting collapsing of that airway

Stabilizing the pharyngeal airway to minimize narrowing and collapse no medications yet exist to stimulate the pharyngeal dilator muscles, and surgery to the soft tissues of the pharynx and tongue is rarely effective (➔ Chapter 11), but mechanical devices are, specifically CPAP and mandibular advancement devices (MADs) (➔ Chapter 10).

Continuous positive airway pressure for obstructive sleep apnoea

The pathogenesis of OSA involves the collapse of the pharyngeal airway (unsupported as it is by bone or cartilage) in response to the negative intraluminal pressure associated with inspiration. CPAP is a treatment that counters this, a pump that generates positive pressure delivered to the pharyngeal airway via a comfortable mask, through the nose (or nose and mouth) producing a 'pneumatic splint'. This seminal advance in the management of OSA came in 1981 with the first report of nasal CPAP providing a pneumatic splint to the pharyngeal airway during sleep. There is high-quality evidence as to benefits on numerous fronts (noted later) but although multiple observational studies have reported reduced mortality, there are no randomized long-term trials to confirm this (➔ see chapter 7 and 8).

Effective use is associated with:
- Reduction or elimination of excessive sleepiness along with a reduction in road traffic accidents, improved productivity, and domestic harmony
- Reduction of elevated blood pressure
- Reduced cardiovascular morbidity
- Improved insulin sensitivity with possible benefits to diabetic control.

Indications for treatment

There are differing, somewhat arbitrary, thresholds for intervening.

The AASM suggests a trial of CPAP in:
- All patients with a RDI of >15, irrespective of symptoms
- Those with a RDI of just >5 and relevant symptoms of sleepiness, insomnia, intrusive snoring, atrial fibrillation, or T2D
- Those with a RDI of >5, irrespective of symptoms in the setting of mission-critical work (commercial road or aviation transport for example) with perhaps the concern about underreporting of sleepiness.

This author, however, has some concerns about this liberal approach. Although not denying that 'if in doubt, pressurize the snout', a more precise interpretation of the respiratory disturbance is in order. Respiratory events contributing to the overall value of the RDI are invariably initially REM sleep related. The clinical impact of these is different from those distributed more evenly throughout the night and their treatment requires a more considered, conservative approach.

The alternative use of the 3% or 4% ODI, typically from overnight pulse oximetry (Fig. 9.1), inevitably underestimates the degree of SDB detected by PSG studies but is pragmatic, though with the same caveat noted earlier.

The additional analysis of pulse rate variability can potentially identify arousals from sleep related to disordered breathing not sufficient to cause significant desaturations, and should be considered in the overall assessment.

Once adherent to treatment, frequency of follow-up is dictated by the symptomatic response, along with objective data including time used, mask leak, and residual AHI. With good control of SDB, an annual review is sufficient.

Repeat sleep testing might be considered to better understand treatment failure and especially to rule out additional sleep pathology such as periodic limb movements.

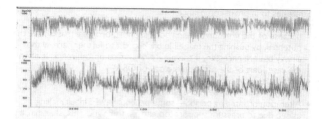

Fig. 9.1 A typical overnight oximetry recording from 22.00 to 05.30 demonstrating repetitive desaturations associated with apnoeas/hypopneas and with commensurate increased pulse rate variability signifying arousals, worse at times consistent with REM sleep, circa 23.30, 01.30, 02.30, and 05.30.

Introduction of CPAP

The machines producing the background positive pressure are 'smart', compensating for leaks and varying pressure needs and need no special adjustments. The nasal or oronasal interface, however, is personal and crucial to acceptance of the treatment. Time spent on this is time well spent.

Problems with CPAP

Patient compliance with this effective treatment is poor. Regular use is generally as low as 50% (compared with 80% reported from some centres perhaps employing fewer trials of CPAP).

What is adequate treatment? An accepted albeit arbitrary standard is >4 hours/night for 5 nights/week. It is appreciated, however, that more is better, with 6 hours/night improving objectively measured sleepiness (the mean sleep latency over four naps being then >7.5 minutes) and 7.5 hours normalizing the Functional Outcome of Sleep Questionnaire.

Note also that compliance is a moving target, with newer machines providing a range of usage options such as:
• Average hours of use per day
• Average hours of use per day used (which itself may be very low).

Adherence may be influenced by the age, sex, and marital/partnership status of the individual as well as socioeconomic and psychological factors. The presenting symptom(s) may also have an impact with insomnia (a feature in 20%) making acceptance less likely than excessive sleepiness (a feature in 45%).

Reasons for poor usage usually relate to problems tolerating the device due to:
• High mask pressures
• Claustrophobia
• Nasal congestion
• Psychological issues
• Lack of initial instruction, or of support, in follow-up.

Strategies to improve compliance:
- Mask fitting—the nasal route is preferable if nasal patency permits because of the firm surrounding bony support; oronasal masks have the potential, by pushing the mandible backwards, to further narrow the airway but are necessary if the nasal airway is compromised as is often the case (part of the pathophysiology of OSA)
- Remote assessment of usage allowing intervention in the first week when remedies may be more effective
- Alteration of ramping period—some patients have difficulty falling asleep due to pressure support too early in the night. This issue may be resolved by extending the period over which the pressure support rises
- Humidification (needed in two-thirds of users)
- Flexible expiratory pressures (pressure relief)
- Bi-level positive airway pressure (i.e. pre-set inspiratory and lower expiratory pressures)—although without formal ratification through controlled studies, this is a strategy most practitioners endorse as worth considering if excessive mask pressure is the problem
- 'Adjuvant' therapy—combining CPAP with a MAD to allow a reduction in mask pressures; an unusual strategy but biologically plausible. Strategies to improve adherence:
- Education, education, education … along with cognitive behavioural therapy a structured psychotherapeutic method altering attitudes and behaviours with efficacy reported in several randomized trials. The consequences of OSA and the beneficial effects of CPAP should be emphasized
- Management of the side effects of CPAP therapy and behavioural therapy seems to be the most reasonable approaches to improve adherence.

Further options for the management of obstructive sleep apnoea

Mandibular advancement devices

(For further details, see ➐ Chapter 10.)

Advanced positioning of the mandible draws the tongue forward to create a larger retroglossal pharyngeal area:

- This may be the preferred treatment in milder cases of OSA and in those whose OSA is largely positional (occurring in the supine sleeping position)
- Studies have also shown a value in patients with more severe OSA who are poorly tolerant of CPAP.

Comparative studies highlight the equivalence of CPAP and MADs related to the longer nightly use of a MAD.

Various types of MADs are available, from the homemade (boil and bite), to mono block (one piece, non-adjustable), to bespoke (adjustable).

Alternative therapies

- Positional therapy—when OSA is predominantly positional, occurring in the supine position, confining sleep to the decubitus position is a rational option using, e.g. a tennis ball stitched into the back of the nightwear, or a proprietary positioning device alerting the user through vibrations, or a MAD
- Head position is a subtle variant, where the head positioned to the side while the patient is supine, leads to obstructive events
- Electrical stimulation—hypoglossal nerve stimulation leads to significant reductions in the AHI and the ODI but requires the surgical implantation of the nerve stimulator (➐ Chapter 12).

Management of central sleep apnoea and obesity hypoventilation syndrome

Consider respiratory support:
- Supplemental O_2 to blunt the hypoxic stimulus to ventilation reduces the AHI by 50%
- CPAP also has a beneficial effect to the same degree, perhaps by reducing afterload on the heart, and/or increasing functional residual lung capacity along with O_2 reserves
- Smart CPAP or adaptive servo-ventilation—varying inspiratory pressures and tidal volumes to stabilize ventilation and therefore CO_2 and saturation, but may be detrimental to those with an ejection fraction of <45%.

For OHS, treatment is by supporting ventilation during sleep through bi-level positive pressure, i.e. non-invasive ventilation, with the expiratory PAP titrated to abolish OSA and the inspiratory PAP to normalize the CO_2.

Further reading

Askland K, Wright L, Wozniak DR, et al. Educational, supportive and behavioural interventions to improve usage of continuous positive airway pressure machines in adults with obstructive sleep apnoea. Cochrane Database Syst Rev. 2020; 4:CD007736.

Gay P, Weaver T, Loube D, Iber C, et al. Evaluation of positive airway pressure treatment for sleep related breathing disorders in adults. Sleep. 2006;29(3):381–401.

Kushida CA, Littner MR, Hirshkowitz M, et al. Practice parameters for the use of continuous and bilevel positive airway pressure devices to treat adult patients with sleep-related breathing disorders. Sleep. 2006;29(3):375–80.

Williams AJ. The sleepy patient. Medicine. 2012;40(6):283–86.

Chapter 10

Dental approaches to the management of sleep-disordered breathing

Aditi Desai

Introduction

Treatment for SDB varies between PAP therapy, which remains the 'gold standard' treatment of choice, oral appliance therapy (OAT), surgery and adjunctive treatments such as weight loss, positional therapy, and emerging alternatives such as genioglossal nerve stimulation.

An appreciation of the high numbers of patients who are either unable to tolerate or unwilling to accept PAP therapy has led to OAT being more widely sought after. These oral appliances have emerged as a viable alternative to PAP therapy. Dental expertise is essential for optimal and delivery of OAT.

Dentistry has always been interested in delivery of OAT for sleep bruxism and temporomandibular joint dysfunction, but emerging evidence indicates the selection of oral appliance may depend on further evaluation of the patient to establish the existence of concomitant SDB.

The role of dentists in sleep medicine involves screening and assessing patients at risk, as well as working with a multidisciplinary team of medical professionals providing essential care with oral appliances for SDB, temporomandibular joint dysfunction, and sleep bruxism, the latter of which has been reclassified as a movement disorder in the ICSD-3.

History of oral appliances

The basic concept of OAT has been well understood for over a century. Through human evolution, the separation of the palate from the epiglottis has left a longer and unsupported airway. The tongue in other mammals sits entirely in the oral cavity but in humans the longer flexible airway allows the tongue to sit partially in the oropharyngeal space. This allows for a soft walled oropharynx, providing for speech but also creating a potential for airway collapse during sleep. Continued evolution has also seen the human facial bone structure change to lie behind the frontal region of the brain.

These evolutionary changes have opened up an area of special interest for dentists, namely dental sleep medicine. The basis of dental sleep medicine is provision of stable oral appliances that activate oropharyngeal soft structures by repositioning of the mandible.

Historically, stabilization of the upper airway was carried out by suturing the tongues of micrognathic infants to the lower lip. By 1930, other types of oral appliances and methods of mandibular repositioning were carried out using chin straps and helmets, but OAT, did not come about until 1934. Subsequently, maxillofacial surgery was reported to advance the mandible and maxilla to improve the airway. In 1982, the first oral appliance for OSA, a tongue retaining device, was introduced by Samuelson.

Oral appliance therapy

Oral appliances have emerged as a viable alternative for treatment of snoring and OSA, for use as an alternative while travelling, or as combination treatment with PAP in patients unable to tolerate high pressures. Despite increasing evidence of efficacy of OAT, barriers to treatment with oral appliances exist. One such barrier has been the time taken to initiate treatment. CPAP can be administered almost immediately and, with remote access, can be titrated from a distance but OAT has conventionally taken at least two or three visits with impression taking, protrusive bite registration, and fitting of device, with additional visits for protrusive adjustment (titration) and dealing with any complications. This aspect of the barrier to treatment will soon be a thing of the past with the advent and use of digital technology and three-dimensional printing. Use of intraoral scanning, telemedicine, and the creation of a digital workflow will mean appliances can in theory be made within a few hours. These may be 'interim' devices for patients who require immediate relief of symptoms while the more robust device is being manufactured.

Treatment predictive factors

The treatment of loud habitual snoring and OSA cannot be guaranteed without proper airway evaluation. Multilevel collapse as well as the different aspects of airway collapse anteroposteriorly, laterally, or concentrically should be assessed to treat the disease effectively and this can only be achieved if dentists collaborate with ENT colleagues.

There are several patient factors that can be assessed in order to establish treatment outcome. Patients are more likely to have a positive outcome with the following criteria:

- Low level of disease, i.e. low AHI or benign snoring
- Low BMI
- Small collar size
- Patients who have supine-dependent OSA are more likely to respond to OAT than lateral sleepers. This is more efficacious using positional therapy in combination with OAT
- Younger age
- Female sex
- Anatomical considerations, such as shorter length of soft palate, lower hyoid bone position, and significant retrognathia. Imaging, drug-induced sleep endoscopy, or awake nasendoscopy using certain manoeuvres may be helpful.

Types of oral appliances

Oral appliances for OSA fall into three broad categories:
- 'Off-the-shelf' self-fit or 'boil-and-bite' devices
- Tongue retaining devices
- Customized or bespoke devices:
  - Mono-bloc or one-piece devices
  - Bi-bloc or two-part adjustable devices.

There are over a hundred oral appliances available globally and each one has its own unique design features. Differences predominantly relate to:

- The degree of customization to the patient's dentition
- One-piece (monobloc) designs with no mouth opening
- Two-piece variants with separate upper and lower components with varying coupling mechanisms.

Two-piece appliances also vary in permissible:
- Lateral jaw movement
- Range of degree of advancement
- Amount of vertical opening
- Fabrication material
- Amount of occlusal coverage.

'Boil-and-bite' devices

These are useful in cases where cost is an issue or when a patient is unable to access a service where a bespoke device can be delivered.

Temporary or trial devices have an important role in the following circumstances while offering the patient some relief:
- Evaluation of the potential success of OAT prior to the cost of a more robust bespoke device
- To give a sceptical patient an opportunity to experience the benefit of OAT. This has to be managed with care as trial devices are not the most comfortable or robust in their application, which may lead to the patient declining treatment
- As a device to achieve the optimum protrusion through incremental titration and using that record to make a monobloc device
- In cases where a patient has lost or fractured the bespoke device.

Tongue retaining devices

These are useful for edentulous patients and used in combination with a bi-bloc device to help advance the tongue further in some patients. They are useful as a trial to establish if the tongue base is the major cause of obstruction. These have not gained in popularity, however, due to short- and long-term complications.

Custom-made appliances

These have two subcategories.

Mono-blocs are a one-piece device usually made of silicone and fitted to a predetermined protrusion of the lower jaw. They can be adequately effective for patients with healthy dentition and mild SDB, but are contraindicated in:
- Patients with sleep bruxism, as inability to continue bruxing leads to complications
- Mouth breathers due to limited air hole anteriorly
- Claustrophobic patients.

Bi-bloc adjustable devices have been shown to be the most effective and well tolerated. These are two components that are effectively coupled to anchor the lower jaw in protrusion to stabilize the distance between hyoid and genioglossal insertion. The mechanism with which this is achieved is unique to each appliance manufacturer.

The ability to move the lower jaw laterally as well as being able to open the mouth vertically (to be able to speak and/or take a sip of water while wearing it) is a feature sought after by patients who should be an integral part of the device selection process.

Mechanism of action of OAT

Oral appliances act to modulate airway anatomy. Tongue retaining devices suction the tongue forward to prevent it from falling back and obstructing the airway during sleep, but most appliances act by modifying the position of the mandible (Fig. 10.1):

- By advancing the mandible, it is generally thought that the increase in oropharyngeal space occurs anteroposteriorly due to the forward movement of the mandible taking the tongue forward with it
- Neuromuscular activity may be the reason for enlargement of the upper airway with an increase in the velopharyngeal space anteroposteriorly and laterally, as demonstrated during magnetic resonance imaging (MRI) and nasendoscopy. This increase in dimension may be the result of various oral structures and muscles that lead to the stretching of the palatoglossal and palatopharyngeal muscles and subsequently the arches
- Stretching of the curvature of the velopharynx has been shown in studies to improve aerodynamics, hence airway resistance
- Stabilization of the mandible and hyoid bone prevents backward and downward rotation of the mandible and relapse of the tongue leading to airway obstruction.

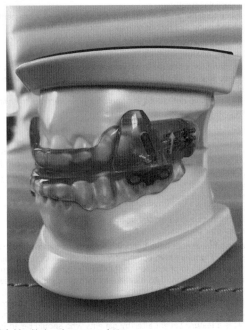

Fig. 10.1 Mandibular advancement device.

Side effects and complications of OAT

As OAT has evolved over the last few decades, side effects of such therapy have also been recognized in increasing numbers. The most significant side effect that concerns patients most is unwanted tooth movement and bite changes. There are other side effects and complications that are reported in the literature:

- Effect on soft tissues and complications of device wear:
  - Hypersalivation
  - Dry mouth
  - Material sensitivity
  - Mucosal and gingival irritation
  - Tongue soreness
  - Anxiety and claustrophobia
  - Gagging
- Damage to teeth and restorations:
  - Tooth for restoration fractures
  - Dislodging of restorations and debonding of extracoronal crowns and bridges
- Temporomandibular joint and accompanying muscle and ligament side effects:
  - Transient jaw pain on device removal
  Tenderness in masticatory muscles
  - Joint sounds such as clicking
  - Pain in the temporomandibular joint which is persistent
- Occlusal changes.

Because of these potential complications, it is important that OAT is overseen by a dentist with specialist expertise in this area. Many of these issues can be monitored for, and addressed. Minimizing or prevention of these side effects enhances patient adherence and optimum treatment outcome. Some of these are more significant than others but should be considered in conjunction with good clinical judgement, weighing the risk versus benefit to the patient when considering remedy of the situation.

Conclusion

An understanding of the criteria for successful OAT, a knowledge of how these appliances work, and how to manage side effects will influence how successful the treatment will be. This is essential to optimize treatment outcome and a positive patient experience.

OAT should be considered as a treatment for mild SDB, or in more severe cases as an adjunct to traditional therapies, where those traditional therapies have been poorly tolerated.

Further reading

British Society for Dental Sleep Medicine. Available at: ℘ https://bsdsm.org.uk/

Clark GT, Blumenfeld I, Yoffe N, et al. A crossover study comparing the efficacy of continuous positive airway pressure with anterior mandibular positioning devices on patients with obstructive sleep apnea. Chest. 1996;109(6):1477–83.

Ferguson KA, Ono T, Lowe AA, et al. A randomized crossover study of an oral appliance vs nasal-continuous positive airway pressure in the treatment of mild-moderate obstructive sleep apnea. Chest. 1996;109(5):1269–75.

Ramar K, Dort LC, Katz SG, et al. Clinical practice guideline for the treatment of obstructive sleep apnea and snoring with oral appliance therapy: an update for 2015. J Clin Sleep Med. 2015;11(7):773–827.

Surgical approaches to the management of sleep-disordered breathing

Bhik Kotecha

Introduction

Sleep-related breathing disorders include patients suffering from primary snoring, upper airway resistance syndrome, and OSA. In these patients, the turbulent airflow from the nose to the larynx is due to various anatomical obstructive segments resulting in snoring and apnoeic episodes.

The otolaryngologist can provide useful input in managing many of these patients presenting with SDB. The standard recommended treatment for moderate and severe OSA is CPAP, but the compliance and adherence of this form of therapy is somewhat poor. These patients could be referred to the otolaryngologist for evaluation and perhaps surgical rectification of the obstructive upper airway, which may result in lowering the pressure requirement for CPAP, thus improving compliance and adherence rates and occasionally may well alleviate the need of CPAP therapy.

Careful patient selection is the key in attaining good surgical outcomes and this certainly applies to patients with SDB. It is important to assess the upper airway carefully and accurately both during wakefulness and while asleep, as the muscle tone and obstructive events would differ in these two states. Assessing the airway during natural physiological sleep is difficult, if not impossible, and therefore the technique of drug-induced sleep endoscopy can be utilized. In general, obese patients with a high BMI fare worse following surgery for SDB as there is extrinsic compression of the upper airway by the parapharyngeal fat space as well as fat deposition in the base of the tongue.

Surgery for SDB can be divided into soft tissue surgery and skeletal framework surgery. Furthermore, depending on the severity of SDB, either minimally invasive surgery or more radical and aggressive surgical intervention may be required.

The role of surgery in SDB can be curative, but more often it is adjunctive and can help compliance with CPAP or oral appliances. Surgical units offering surgery for severe SDB patients need good support from the anaesthetic department and the infrastructure of their hospital has to be such so as to nurse them in a high dependency unit.

Clinical evaluation of the upper airway

Clinical evaluation commences with inspection of the skeletal framework followed by a thorough assessment of the internal aspect of the upper airway (Fig. 11.1) using a fibreoptic flexible nasopharyngoscope:

Skeletal framework

- External nasal bone deformity
- Retrognathia
- Maxillary retrusion.

Nose and nasal cavity

- Anatomical:
  - Nasal valve deformity
  - Deviated nasal septum
  - Hypertrophy of inferior turbinate
- Physiological:
  - Vasomotor rhinitis
  - Allergic rhinitis
- Pathological:
  - Nasal polyposis
  - Rhinosinusitis.

Oral cavity

- Limited mouth opening
- Size of tonsils
- Soft palate—length, thickness, and general laxity
- Uvula—thickness and length.

Tongue base and larynx

- Lymphoid hyperplasia or muscular hypertrophy
- Reduced retroglossal dimension
- Mallampati and Friedman tongue position status
- Floppy epiglottis
- Laryngeal pathology
- Acid reflux.

Awake and asleep assessment

The upper airway collapse seen during sleep is very different compared to what is observed during wakefulness.

With the nasopharyngoscope in position, the patient can be asked to simulate snoring sounds to assess the vibrations of the soft palate and to perform the Müller's manoeuvre to ascertain the degree of obstruction at various levels of the pharyngeal lumen. This manoeuvre essentially involves a reversed Valsalva with the endoscope in position in the pharynx. When the endoscope is within the lumen of the pharynx, the patient is instructed to breathe in and suck simultaneously with the mouth closed and nostrils pinched. One can then determine what anatomical segment causes the most potential obstruction.

This awake evaluation could give a false impression of the dynamics of the upper airway obstruction when compared to nocturnal events. For this reason, drug-induced sleep endoscopy has gained popularity and is performed with the help of an anaesthetist to induce sleep by administrating propofol with or without midazolam. The depth of sedation can be controlled by using bispectral index monitoring, a tool commonly used by anaesthetists which essentially reflects EEG activity and gives a rough idea as to how deeply the patient is sedated. During the procedure, the proportion of involvement of different anatomical segments of the pharyngeal lumen is noted, thus guiding what surgical procedure is appropriate at each level.

Recent evidence suggests that dynamic sleep MRI may also provide a reliable technique for the characterization of the site of airway obstruction.

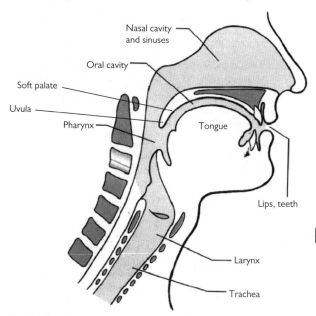

Fig. 11.1 Sagittal section of the upper airway illustrating the naso-pharynx, oro-pharynx and the hypo-pharynx.

Surgical procedures for sleep-disordered breathing

A variety of surgical procedures are available to correct different regions of the obstructive upper airway. Techniques using radiofrequency probes have been innovated to address the nasal turbinates, soft palate, and the base of the tongue. Radiofrequency technology is less aggressive than the previously popular laser and is preferred particularly in the less severe SDB. Radiofrequency technique applies heat energy interstitially and thus for the nasal turbinates and base of the tongue results in reduction of tissue volume, thus creating more space, and in the soft palate changes the mechanical properties of the elastic fibres, creating more stiffening of the palate. The cutting needle can be used to shorten the soft palate simultaneously.

For less severe SDB, if the region of obstruction is the soft palate, then techniques such as injection sclerotherapy, pillar implants, or simple interstitial radiofrequency thermotherapy would suffice and attains a more stiffened soft palate without altering the shape of the palate.

However, if SDB is more severe, then excision of the redundant palate–pharyngeal mucosa may be required thus resulting in a slightly altered shape of the palate. Naturally, great care has to be taken to avoid complications such as nasal regurgitation by being conservative while resecting the amount of soft palate tissue.

Further developments in palatal surgery have entailed relocation of the palatopharyngeus muscle to the hamulus.

Skeletal framework surgery is more aggressive but attains very good surgical outcomes in carefully selected individuals undergoing maxillomandibular advancement surgery.

Nose
- Nasal septoplasty (correction of deviated nasal septum)
- Septorhinoplasty
- Functional endoscopic sinus surgery
- Nasal polypectomy
- Turbinate reduction or turbinoplasty.

Oropharyngeal surgery
- Tonsillectomy/tonsillotomy
- Palatoplasty (various modifications of uvulopharyngoplasty)
- Palatal pillar implants
- Injection palatal sclerotherapy
- Interstitial radiofrequency to soft palate.

Hypopharyngeal surgery
- Radiofrequency ablation
- Midline glossectomy
- Genioglossus advancement
- Hyoid suspension
- Epiglottic wedge resection.

Skeletal framework surgery
- Geniotubercle advancement
- Mandibular osteotomy
- Maxillomandibular advancement.

Recent advances in surgery for sleep-disordered breathing

In the last couple of decades, great attempts have been made to improve surgical outcomes for SDB and this has been made possible by increasing the meticulous manner in which the upper airway obstruction has been evaluated, particularly since the innovation of drug-induced sleep endoscopy. Furthermore, this has been complemented by advances in technology to attain less thermal trauma to the soft tissue with the introduction of radiofrequency technology.

The innovation of transoral robotic surgery has made the challenging task of addressing the obstructive hypopharynx a lot easier and now is not uncommonly utilized in patients who have failed CPAP therapy and have a significant hypopharyngeal obstruction secondary to a very prominent base of tongue and/or epiglottis. This improves the laryngeal inlet and thus relieves the upper airway obstruction.

Finally, in the last decade, the introduction of the techniques utilizing hypoglossal nerve stimulation (➲ Chapter 12) has brought hope for the very challenging cases of SDB patients who have failed all other possible treatment modalities.

Long-term successful outcome in these patients selected by drug-induced sleep endoscopy evaluation has been reported.

Further reading

Camacho M, Riaz M, Capasso R, et al. The effect of nasal surgery on continuous positive airway pressure device use and therapeutic treatment pressures: a systematic review and meta-analysis. Sleep. 2015;38(2):279–86.

Gamaleldin O, Bhagat A, Anwar O, et al. Role of dynamic sleep MRI in obstructive sleep apnoea syndrome. Oral Radiol. 2021;37(3):376–84.

Lechner M, Wilkins D, Kotecha B. A review on drug induced sedation endoscopy – technique, grading systems and controversies. Sleep Med Rev. 2018;41:414–18.

Sethukumar P, Kotecha B. Tailoring surgical interventions to treat obstructive sleep apnoea: one size does not fit all. Breathe. 2018;14(3):e84–93.

Strollo PJ Jr, Soose RJ, Mauer JT, et al. Upper-airway stimulation for obstructive sleep apnea. N Engl J Med. 2014;370(2):139–49.

Virk JS, Kotecha B. Otorhinolaryngological aspects of sleep-related breathing disorders. J Thorac Dis 2016;8(2):213–23.

Novel approaches for the treatment of obstructive sleep apnoea

Joerg Steier

Introduction

Standard therapy for SDB is effective and well established. Most commonly, CPAP therapy is used for the treatment of moderate to severe OSA (➔ Chapter 9), while mild OSA can be treated using a MAD (➔ Chapter 10) dental physicians (➔ chapter 9).

CPAP therapy restores upper airway patency while asleep, avoids sleep fragmentation, improves daytime functioning and sleepiness, and, potentially, improves long-term cardiovascular risks associated with SDB. However, CPAP therapy requires good compliance. Patients need to sleep with a mask, either full-face, nasal, or mouth, to transmit the pressures. This is an ongoing treatment, as OSA returns when patients no longer use CPAP. Long-term compliance in OSA is limited—within the first 6 weeks of treatment, a quarter of patients struggle to make sufficient use of it and after 1 year, about half of the patients who should be treated use CPAP in a way that provides no therapeutic effect.

Alternative treatment options for OSA are therefore required. The following departments may provide further support in selecting suitable novel therapeutic approaches:

* Respiratory physicians
* ENT surgeons (➔ Chapter 11)
* Bariatric services
* Maxillofacial surgeons.

Electrical stimulation

In recent years, the revival of electrical stimulation of the dilator muscles of the upper airway has seen a renaissance. Early attempts to use electrical current in the submental area caused pain and woke patients, but more recent trials have used lower current and longer stimulation periods to sustain neuromuscular tone of the upper airway following sleep onset.

Transcutaneous electrical stimulation of the upper airway has been used in physiological studies to maintain upper airway patency while asleep. It has been shown to:

* Reduce the AHI
* Reduce the RDI
* Reduce snoring
* Increase oxygenation
* Reduce work of breathing
* Reduce neural respiratory drive.

Transcutaneous electrical stimulation: a randomized controlled trial

In a recent randomized and sham-controlled cross-over trial (Continuous Transcutaneous Electrical Stimulation in Sleep Apnoea (TESLA) trial, NCT01661712), it was shown that transcutaneous electrical stimulation can be delivered throughout the night, improve sleep apnoea, and be tolerated without significant adverse effects.

The TESLA trial revealed that nocturnal transcutaneous electrical stimulation in OSA:
- Improves the oxygen desaturation index (4% ODI, primary outcome parameter)
- Improves the AHI in responders
- Improves the arousal index and N1 modestly.

Treatment effects were modest for 'all-comers', but highly significant in a selected subgroup of responders who were slim and with mild to moderate OSA.

The treatment effect was modest, but in responders to the stimulation (47%) the effect was significant in that OSA severity was improved. Responders to this treatment are defined as someone whose:
- AHI improves by at least >50% and to an AHI below 20/hour
- ODI improves by at least 25% and to an ODI below 20/hour
- AHI and ODI improve back to normal (<5/hour).

The treatment did not have any significant adverse events or side effects; patients felt that their dry mouth improved with electrical stimulation.

Successful use of transcutaneous electrical stimulation depends on:
- Current intensity
- Frequency
- Wave shape
- Pauses
- Titration to comfort.

Hypoglossal nerve stimulation: a randomized controlled trial

The implantation of a hypoglossal nerve stimulator on the right side had been tested in previous studies and in 2014, the results of a randomized, treatment withdrawal controlled trial were published (Stimulation Therapy for Apnea Reduction (STAR) trial, NCT01161420).

Patients with an AHI between 20 and 50/hour were included and pre-assessed by ENT surgeons using drug-induced sleep endoscopy. Patients with concentric or multilevel obstruction were found to be less likely to respond to the treatment and excluded from the study.

The STAR trial proved that hypoglossal nerve stimulation led to:
Improved AHI
- Improved ODI
- Reduced effects of sleep apnoea (percentage of time with oxygen saturation <90%)
- Improved quality of life (FOSQ, Epworth Sleepiness Scale)
- There was a low rate of procedure-related serious adverse events of 2%.

Treatment effects were well preserved at 12 months and, recently, the 5-year follow-up data on the initial cohort were published, revealing an on-going treatment effect with good compliance.

According to the National Institute for Health and Care Excellence (NICE) in the UK, hypoglossal nerve stimulation may have the following adverse effects:
- Transient ipsilateral hemi-tongue paresis
- Tongue abrasion
- Bleeding
- Rupture of a vein
- Seroma
- Headache
- Infection
- Dry mouth
- Discomfort due to stimulation
- Paraesthesiae
- Device migration
- Device removal due to insomnia, septic joint infection, and non-response
- Leads breaking
- Defective implanted pulse-generator connector
- Other complications including pain, stiffness, sore throat, stitch abscess, local swelling, fever, and lack of tongue response to stimulation
- Theoretical adverse events included fatigue of the muscles and hypoglossal nerve damage.

Ongoing studies and clinical trials

There are currently ongoing trials by different providers with specific adjustments to try and refine the invasive or non-invasive use of electrical stimulation for OSA:

- Inspire®: following the STAR trial, the system has been approved in the US, Germany, and other countries; there is ongoing recruitment for the post-approval study, the adherence and outcome registry and a trial using this method in Down syndrome (see I in Fig. 12.1)
- ImThera®: this system uses targeted unilateral hypoglossal nerve stimulation (see II in Fig. 12.1)
- Nyxoah®: this system uses a median approach with a mounted external energy source for bilateral hypoglossal nerve stimulation (see III in Fig. 12.1)
- TESLA/TESLA home: these are the only non-commercial trials testing transcutaneous electrical stimulation in sleep apnoea. Following the initial trial, TESLA home will soon open for the use of domiciliary transcutaneous electrical stimulation (see blue square in Fig. 12.1).

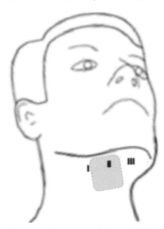

Fig. 12.1 Location of hypoglossal nerve stimulation according to different methods (see text); I and II with a unilateral, and III with a median and bilateral approach to transcutaneous electrical stimulation.

Future research

The use of electrical stimulation for the treatment of OSA requires further investigations to continue to optimize clinical use. The following specifications need to be selected to tailor individual efficiency and comfort:

* Current intensity and duration
* Location of stimulation site
* Unilateral versus bilateral stimulation
* Stimulation pattern (triggered, intermittent, continuous)
* Target muscles and optimal titration.

Clinical efficacy and long-term outcomes as well as cost-efficiency are currently being tested in ongoing clinical trials. Implications for cardiovascular comorbidity and usage in patients who are not self-caring with CPAP therapy are a different focus of future studies. Adverse events have been well described and post-market experience is permanently audited.

Patient and public involvement

Patient and public involvement has been published in this field. Patients with OSA have been asked to feed back on the techniques after being shown, and the methods explained, CPAP and MADs as established treatments. They were further shown pictures and the methodologies of hypoglossal nerve and transcutaneous electrical stimulation in OSA were explained. They ranked their preference in the following order, highest first:
Transcutaneous electrical stimulation

* Hypoglossal nerve stimulation
* CPAP
* MADs.

These results underline the importance to develop further alternative treatment options for OSA despite existing efficient treatment modalities.

NICE guidance

NICE undertook a public consultation that resulted in an interventional procedures guidance (IPG598) in 2017 with the following recommendations:

* Current experience on hypoglossal nerve stimulation is limited in quantity and quality
* The procedure should only be used with special arrangements for clinical governance, consent, and audit or research
* Clinicians need to inform their clinical governance leads, inform patients sufficiently about current limitations, and audit and review clinical outcomes
* Patient selection and procedure should be undertaken by clinicians with special expertise
* Further research including the use of observational data from registries should provide information on patient selection, safety outcomes, quality of life, long-term outcomes, and the value of the procedure in the treatment pathway.

Further alternatives

Other alternative treatment options for OSA may include more potent ventilatory support or other surgical options:

- Weight loss and weight loss surgery
- Non-invasive ventilation, triggered bi-level ventilation is commonly described as more comfortable and easier to tolerate as it synchronizes with the patient's respiratory effort. It is potent enough to treat OSA and could improve compliance in selected cases
- In CSA, different ventilator modes (adaptive servo-ventilation) have been developed to adjust to the respiratory pattern and avoid apnoeic episodes. However, the Treatment of Predominant Central Sleep Apnoea by Adaptive Servo Ventilation in Patients With Heart Failure (SERVE-HF) trial using this method observed that patients with reduced ejection fraction had a higher mortality than the control group
- Surgical intervention with nasal obstruction
- Upper throat surgery on palate, tonsils, and/or uvula (e.g. uvulopalatopharyngoplasty)
- Structural skeletal procedures to extend the palate or the maxilla, in some cases a maxilla–mandibular advancement might be indicated
- In some countries, modafinil is used for treating residual sleepiness. Solriamfetol is another agent currently being assessed for this indication
- Experimental combinations of medications are currently trialled in laboratory-based experiments to target sleep apnoea mechanisms and may in future lead to additionally available treatments.

There is good evidence for the efficacy of weight loss, if indicated. However, there is limited evidence for efficacy, cost-effectiveness, and long-term outcomes for the other listed treatments in the context of sleep apnoea.

Further reading

Bisogni V, Pengo MF, De Vito A, et al. Electrical stimulation for the treatment of obstructive sleep apnoea: a review of the evidence. Expert Rev Respir Med. 2017;11(9):711–20.

He B, Al-Sherif M, Nido M, et al. Domiciliary use of transcutaneous electrical stimulation for patients with obstructive sleep apnoea: a conceptual framework for the TESLA home programme. J Thorac Dis. 2019;11(5):2153–64.

Pengo MF, Steier J. Emerging technology: electrical stimulation in obstructive sleep apnoea. J Thorac Dis. 2015;7(8):1286–97.

Restless legs syndrome and periodic limb movement disorder

Guy Leschziner

Introduction

Restless legs syndrome (RLS) is a neurological disorder that often goes un-diagnosed and untreated, despite its frequency. This is in part due to the variability in its presentation and consequences for sleep, causing both sleep initiation and sleep maintenance issues. However, until recently its very existence as a condition has been subject to debate, despite a wealth of clinical, genetic, biochemical, and pathological evidence to the contrary. An awareness of this disorder is fundamental to the practice of medicine in a number of specialties and general practice.

Definition

RLS is a common neurological disorder characterized by an urge to move the body, usually but not invariably the legs, often accompanied by a range of unpleasant sensations. In addition to the sensory symptoms, it is a common and frequently unrecognized cause of insomnia, especially sleep initiation difficulties.

RLS is defined by a number of mandatory diagnostic criteria:
- The urge to move body parts, usually legs, accompanied by uncomfortable or unpleasant sensations
- Symptoms start during periods of immobility or sleep, and worsen with immobility
- Movement of the affected limbs results in partial or transient relief
- Symptoms worsen in the evening and night
- The above-listed symptoms are not solely accounted for by another medical condition.

Additional supportive criteria include:
- A family history of RLS in first-degree relatives
- A response to treatment with dopaminergic drugs
- The presence of periodic limb movements of sleep (PLMS).

PLMS occur in up to 90% of patients with RLS. These movements are characterized by involuntary movements of the legs, usually in sleep although occasionally spilling over into wakefulness (periodic limb movements of wakefulness (PLMW)). The leg movements typically involve extension of the hallux, dorsiflexion, flexion of the knee, and flexion of the hip, although sometimes these movements are very subtle.

PLMS are defined as:
- Movements lasting 0.5–5 seconds
- Occurring of intervals of 5–90 seconds
- At least four movements in a series.

PLMS frequently occur in the absence of RLS symptoms however, and are commonly seen as incidental findings on PSG. They are classed as periodic limb movement disorder (PLMD) if they result in frequent arousals from sleep resulting in either unrefreshing sleep, sleep maintenance difficulties, or daytime symptoms such as excessive daytime sleepiness or cognitive dysfunction.

Epidemiology

- RLS prevalence is uncertain but estimates range between 2% and 15% of adults
- It is well described in children, but prevalence increases with age
- Associated conditions include:
  - Pregnancy (up to 26% of women)
  - Iron deficiency
  - Uraemia
  - Peripheral neuropathy, especially small fibre
  - Myelopathy due to multiple sclerosis, syringomyelia, or cord tumours
  - Other neurological disorders such as Parkinson's disease, spinocerebellar ataxias, and essential tremor
- The prevalence of PLMD is unknown, since it requires PSG to ascertain. PLMS are seen in a third of patients over the age of 60 years.

Clinical features

The diagnosis of RLS is usually straightforward, provided the clinician is aware of the entity. However, identification of the clinical features can sometimes be problematic:

- Descriptions of the sensory symptoms can vary greatly. Terms used by patients include a pulling sensation, jittering, itching, bubbling, insects under the skin, electric sensations, tightness, throbbing, and tingling
- RLS can present with predominant pain
- While the legs are the commonest anatomical site affected, RLS can involve the arms, abdomen, chest, genitalia, or face
- Patients may present simply with sleep initiation insomnia, and only a careful history will identify the presence of RLS symptoms.

Isolated PLMD in the absence of RLS symptoms can be much more difficult to diagnose. The bed partner may complain of the patient twitching or jerking in sleep, and one of the commonest presentations is unrefreshing sleep or sleep maintenance issues. Occasionally, a patient report of leg movements in the evening (PLMW) can be very helpful. Patients with PLMD may complain of daytime tiredness or fatigue, but frequently do not complain of profound daytime sleepiness, hence it is often confused with a fatigue syndrome, depression, or other sleep disorders.

Pathophysiology

The pathophysiological basis of RLS/PLMD is not fully elucidated. However, the most widely accepted hypothesis is based upon evidence of alterations in dopaminergic transmission. Evidence points to upregulation of dopamine levels in the substantia nigra, coupled with postsynaptic dopamine receptor downregulation, resulting in alteration of spinal network activity. Iron is an important cofactor in the production of dopamine, hence the role of iron deficiency in the aetiology of RLS, and iron supplementation in its treatment.

There is also a strong genetic component to the aetiology of RLS. Twin studies demonstrate heritability estimates of 50–80%, and genome-wide association studies have identified variants in several genes that are linked to RLS (and PLMS).

Management

It is important to stress that the majority of patients (85%) with RLS and PLMD do not require pharmacological treatment. Prior to initiating medication, efforts should be undertaken to exclude underlying causes:

- Identify behaviours that may exacerbate RLS (e.g. sleep restriction, alcohol, caffeine, nicotine)
- Withdrawal, if possible, of drugs that may trigger or cause RLS:
  - Dopa-blocking agents (e.g. neuroleptics and antiemetics)
  - Beta-blockers and calcium channel antagonists
  - Antihistamines
  - Antidepressant drugs
- Neurological examination
- Renal profile, to exclude uraemia
- Iron studies, especially ferritin. If ferritin <75 micrograms/L, the patient should be commenced on oral iron supplementation.

Non-pharmacological therapies include:
- Optimization of sleep hygiene and consideration of CBT-I
- Relaxation therapy
- Walking or stretching prior to bed
- Massage of affected body parts
- Warm bath prior to bed
- Magnesium supplementation (anecdotal).

Pharmacological therapies should be reserved for those patients in whom the symptoms are having a significant impact on sleep or quality of life, and who have not responded to non-pharmacological measures.

- Dopamine receptor agonists (ropinirole, pramipexole, rotigotine) are licensed for RLS. Common side effects include nausea, grogginess, and postural hypotension. However, dopamine receptor agonists have special considerations:
  - Augmentation: this class of drugs, especially at higher doses, can cause a worsening of RLS beyond that expected from the natural history. This can cause a worsening of the intensity of the symptoms, less relief from movement, symptoms coming on earlier in the day, and spread to different body parts. For this reason, the dose should be maintained at the minimum to adequately control symptoms, and should not be increased beyond a certain threshold (ropinirole 2 mg daily, pramipexole 500 micrograms daily, rotigotine 4 mg daily). Levodopa should not be utilized except for rare 'as-needed' usage, due to extremely high rates of augmentation
  - Impulse control disorders: dopa agonists are associated with reward dysregulation, causing issues such as compulsive eating, gambling, shopping, and hypersexuality, and should be used cautiously in patients with a previous history of substance abuse or psychopathology. All patients should be warned regarding these potential side effects prior to initiation of this class of drugs
- Alpha-2-delta ligands, i.e. gabapentin and pregabalin (both unlicensed): these drugs do not cause impulse control disorders or augmentation, and are helpful in treating sleep fragmentation. Maximum night-time doses are pregabalin 300 mg and gabapentin 900 mg

- Clonazepam: this is a standard (unlicensed) treatment for RLS, particularly if there is prominent comorbid insomnia. The starting dose is typically 0.25–0.5 mg at night
- Opioids: Targinact® (licensed for severe refractory RLS), and other unlicensed treatments such as codeine and tramadol can be particularly helpful for painful leg variant RLS. Methadone has been used in extreme cases to good effect
- Intravenous iron: there is increasing evidence that in some patients with RLS, there is an abnormality of transport of iron across the blood–brain barrier, causing brain deficiency of iron even in the context of normal peripheral markers of iron storage. Intravenous iron is increasingly being utilized in selected patients with refractory RLS.

The management of PLMD in the absence of RLS is less evidence based, and there are no licensed treatments for isolated PLMD. As previously stated, PLMs in sleep are not necessarily associated with sleep complaints, but if there is prominent sleep maintenance insomnia or daytime sequelae, most sleep physicians would treat with the treatments previously listed, as per RLS guidelines. However, many clinicians would favour options that are more sedating, such as the alpha-2-delta ligands or clonazepam.

Further reading

For patients

RLS-UK. Available at: ℬ https://www.rls-uk.org/

For clinicians

Allen RP, Picchietti DL, Auerbach M, et al. Evidence-based and consensus clinical practice guidelines for the iron treatment of restless legs syndrome/Willis-Ekbom disease in adults and children: an IRLSSG task force report. Sleep Med. 2018;41:27–44.

Garcia-Borreguero D, Kohnen R, Silber MH, et al. The long-term treatment of restless legs syndrome/Willis-Ekbom disease: evidence-based guidelines and clinical consensus best practice guidance: a report from the International restless legs syndrome Study Group. Sleep Med. 2013;14(7):675–84.

Garcia-Borreguero D, Stillman P, Benes H, et al. Algorithms for the diagnosis and treatment of restless legs syndrome in primary care. BMC Neurol. 2011;11:28.

Garcia-Borreguero D, Silber MH, Winkelman JW, et al. Guidelines for the first-line treatment of restless legs syndrome/Willis-Ekbom disease, prevention and treatment of dopaminergic augmentation: a combined task force of the IRLSSG, EURLSSG, and the RLS-foundation. Sleep Med. 2016;21:1–11.

Leschziner G, Gringras P. Restless legs syndrome. BMJ. 2012;344:e3056.

Narcolepsy

Panagis Drakatos

Introduction

Narcolepsy is a chronic neurological disorder characterized by excessive daytime sleepiness (EDS) and features of REM-sleep dissociation. It affects ~1 in 2000 people, and it may take up to 10–15 years from the onset of symptoms until the diagnosis is made. According to the ICSD-3, narcolepsy type 1 (NT1) and narcolepsy type 2 (NT2) have replaced the previous diagnostic groups of narcolepsy with or without cataplexy, respectively. The primary reason is the well pathophysiologically defined and homogeneous group of NT1 patients who suffer from low or absent hypocretin-1 (orexin) in the cerebrospinal fluid (CSF) irrespective of the presence of cataplexy.

Narcolepsy type 1

NT1 is considered a chronic neurological disease with specific aetiology (extensive loss of hypothalamic neurons that produce the neuropeptides orexin A and B) and homogeneous clinical and polysomnographic features. EDS is the cardinal symptom, along with REM-sleep dissociation features (intrusion of typical REM phenomena into wakefulness), the most specific of which is cataplexy.

Clinical presentation

- The four cardinal clinical features:
  - *Persistent EDS*: a mandatory feature
  - *Cataplexy*: the intrusion of REM-related partial or complete muscle atonia of voluntary muscles (e.g. facial muscles, limbs, or whole body) into wakefulness, usually in response to an emotional positive or negative stimulus (e.g. laughter, surprise, anger, frustration). Frequency can vary from several events in a day to extremely rarely, and usually lasts seconds to a few minutes. Patients retain consciousness with full recollection of the event afterwards, and deep tendon reflexes are typically absent, especially during full-body cataplexy
  - *Sleep paralysis*: the intrusion of REM-related muscle atonia (usually whole body) into wakefulness, at the beginning, during an arousal, or at the end of the sleep period. The event can last several minutes and can be distressing, with the patient reporting inability to move and talk, often with a feeling of subjective breathlessness. It can also occur up to 20% in the normal population
  - *Hypnagogic and hypnopompic hallucinations*: represent intrusion of the typical REM dreaming state into wakefulness, or in other words dreaming in the awake state, either at the beginning or the end of the sleep period respectively. They can include auditory, visual, and tactile phenomena, but they are less complex or 'fixed' compared to those in patients with psychotic disorders. Similar to sleep paralysis, they usually last up to a couple of minutes and can occur in 20% of the normal population
- Disturbed sleep with increased light sleep (non-REM sleep stage 1)
- Brief naps lasting minutes are usually refreshing
- Other common concomitant sleep disorders: RBD (dream enactment during REM sleep), OSA, PLMS
- Obesity: BMI ~15% above average in adults
- Depression, anxiety: the cause of associated psychological symptoms is unclear. They may relate to the impact of the condition on quality of life, or may be secondary to neurochemical changes seen in narcolepsy.

Demographics

- Prevalence is estimated at 1 per 2000–4000 people (0.025–0.05%) worldwide. In Japan, the prevalence is 1 per 600 people, while in Israel it is 1 per 500,000
- Bimodal distribution of age of onset: peak at ~15 years of age and a smaller peak between 30 and 40 years of age
- Both sexes are affected equally.

Pathophysiology

Current evidence supports an autoimmune process which specifically targets the hypocretin-producing neurons (low or undetectable hypocretin/orexin) in the lateral hypothalamus, in individuals with a genetic susceptibility (human leucocyte antigen (HLA)-DQB1*06:02) that is enhanced by an environmental factor (e.g. infection, H1N1 vaccine).

- Low (<110 pg/mL) or undetectable levels of hypocretin-1 (orexin-A) in CSF
- >98% of patients with NT1 carry HLA-DQB1*06:02 type (12–30% in the general population)
- Seasonal predominance of onset in the symptoms of NT1 in the spring following winter infections
- High titres of antibodies against antistreptolysin O found at the onset of NT1
- Increase of new NT1 cases following administration of a specific brand of vaccine against H1N1 (Pandemrix®).

Diagnostic criteria

According to the ICSD-3, NT1 can be diagnosed when criteria 1 and 2 are met (Table 14.1):

1. Daily periods of irrepressible need to sleep or daytime lapses into sleep, for at least 3 months
2. The presence of one or both of the following:
   - Cataplexy and MSLT shows a MSL ≤8 minutes and ≥2 sleep-onset REM periods (SOREMPs, REM periods within 15 minutes of sleep onset), (1 SOREMP can be replaced with a SOREMP in the preceding PSG)
   - CSF hypocretin-1 concentration is either ≤110 pg/mL or less than one-third of the mean values obtained in normal subjects with the same assay.

The MSLT must be performed immediately after overnight PSG confirming 6 hours of sleep, and be preceded by at least 1 week of actigraphy or sleep diary which will assist in deciding if sleep deprivation, shift work, or another circadian sleep disorder is affecting the results. Patients should also be off drugs that affect sleep for at least 14 days prior to the MSLT and this should be confirmed with a urine drug test. In addition to the PSG features of narcolepsy such as early-onset REM and loss of REM atonia, the overnight study enables the identification of sleep comorbidities that require treatment. See Fig. 14.1.

Treatment

- Sleep hygiene advice
- Scheduled naps can be very beneficial to battle EDS, although pharmacotherapy is usually also required
- Liaison with educational authorities should be offered, and provided with patient agreement. Many patients benefit from individual invigilation during exams, to watch for evidence of sleepiness, and should be given the opportunity to take breaks for short naps if necessary

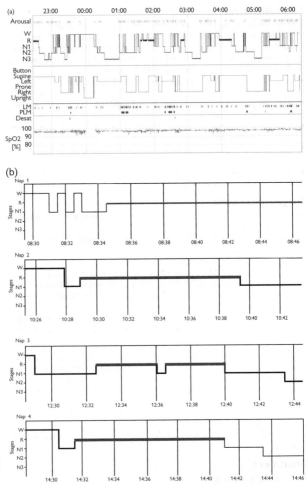

Fig. 14.1 Typical PSG and MSLT of a 26-year-old female patient with NT1. Top figure depicts the PSG which shows early sleep and REM (thick line) onset (SOREMP on nocturnal PSG), with disturbed sleep. Some limb movements are present with an overall normal periodic limb movement index of 9.1 events/hour, and no significant SDB was found with an AHI of 1.0 events/hour. Bottom figure depicts the MSL graph with four SOREMPs out of all 4 naps, all arising from stage 1 sleep as an indicator of increased REM pressure and quick transition from sleep onset to REM sleep. Mean sleep latency was measured at 1.6 minutes fulfilling the criteria for objectively recorded EDS.

- Advice regarding lifestyle and driving. Patients with narcolepsy are usually allowed to drive again when there has been satisfactory symptom control, and depending on the case, satisfactory objective assessment of maintained wakefulness may be required. Regular reviews are required
- Stimulants that help increase alertness and wakefulness:
  - Modafinil (100–400 mg/day in one or two doses, with latest dose before 2 pm; common side effects: headache, anxiety, palpitations, nausea)
  - Amphetamines such as methylphenidate and dexamfetamine (10–60 mg/day in two or three divided doses, or once daily with prolonged-release methylphenidate; common side effects: anxiety, mood swings, nausea)
  - Solriamfetol: is a wake promoter, still under appraisal in UK (75–150mg in the morning; common side effects: headache, nausea, decreased appetite and anxiety)
- Anticataplectic agents that restrict REM sleep. These are also useful in the management of sleep paralysis and hypnagogic hallucinations:
  - Tricyclic antidepressants like clomipramine and imipramine (10–75 mg/day at bedtime; common side effects: antimuscarinic side effects, postural hypotension, confusion, sedation)
  - Reuptake inhibitor medications like venlafaxine (37.5–75 mg twice daily or 37.5–150 mg/day of an extended-release formulation in the morning; common side effects: nausea, headache, insomnia) or fluoxetine (20–60 mg/day in the morning; common side effects: nausea, dry mouth, insomnia)
- Sodium oxybate: is effective for the treatment of both cataplexy and EDS and in the UK is reserved for severe refractory cases (2.25–4.5 g at bedtime and an additional 2.25–4.5 g 2.5–4 hours later; common side effects: nausea, mood swings, and enuresis)
- Pitolisant: is effective for the treatment of both cataplexy and EDS (9–36 mg in the morning; common side effects: anxiety, dizziness, dyspepsia)
- Occasionally patients with very fragmented sleep need pharmacological therapy with sedatives to consolidate night-time sleep.

Differential diagnosis

NT1 is exclusively characterized by cataplexy and low CSF hypocretin-1, and so the presence of either of these features is diagnostic, but:
- It is important to differentiate cataplexy from pseudo-cataplexy, which can occur in normal individuals while laughing out loud or cases of hypotension, or psychological disorders. True cataplexy is usually frequent and triggered by emotions, lasting from a few seconds to minutes, with retained consciousness and recollection of the events by the patient, along with absent deep tendon reflexes during the event. In cases of diagnostic doubt, HLA-DQB1*06:02 and CSF-hypocretin-1 can be measured
- Other sleep disorders (e.g. insufficient sleep syndrome, idiopathic hypersomnia, OSA, PLMS, shift work, and other circadian sleep disorders) or mental conditions, drug misuse, and chronic fatigue syndrome can cause EDS, and some of those early REM onset on nocturnal PSG/MSLT too, but the presence of true cataplexy or low hypocretin-1 would secure the diagnosis of NT1.

Table 14.1 Diagnostic criteria of the major central disorders of hypersomnolence

Diagnostic criteria	NT1	NT2	IH	KLS
Clinical	EDS (*daily*) ≥3 months Cataplexy	EDS (*daily*) ≥3 months Absent cataplexy	EDS (*daily*) ≥3 months Absent cataplexy	≥2 episodes of EDS (*2–35 days each*) ≥1 episode within 18 months Normal between episodes: alertness, cognitive function, behaviour, and mood During episodes ≥1 of cognitive dysfunction, altered perception, eating disorder, and disinhibited behaviour
Sleep study	MSL ≤8 min and ≥2 SOREMPs	MSL ≤8 min and ≥2 SOREMPs	<2 SOREMPs MSL ≤8 min or regular TST of ≥12 hours in 24 hours Sleep deprivation is ruled out	
Laboratory	CSF hcrt-1 ≤110 pg/mL or <1/3 of the mean values obtained in normal subjects with the same assay	CSF hcrt-1 >110 pg/mL or >1/3 of the mean values obtained in normal subjects with the same assay		
Overall		Not better explained by another condition or drugs/ medications	Not better explained by another condition or drugs/ medications	Not better explained by another condition or drugs/ medications

CSF hcrt-1, cerebrospinal fluid hypocretin-1 level; EDS, excessive daytime sleepiness; IH, idiopathic hypersomnia; KLS, Kleine–Levin syndrome; MSL, mean sleep latency; NT1, narcolepsy type 1; NT2, narcolepsy type 2; SOREMPs, sleep-onset REM periods; TST, total sleep time.

Narcolepsy type 2

Narcolepsy type 2 (NT2) is considered a chronic neurological disease that shares PSG features, and many of the clinical features, with NT1. Cataplexy is absent and CSF hypocretin-1 levels should not have been proven to be low. It has no specific aetiology, although some are likely to share the same aetiology as NT1, and may proceed to develop cataplexy and a low CSF-hypocretin subsequently.

Clinical presentation

Similar to NT1 but cataplexy events are absent. If cataplexy events develop over time, then the diagnosis becomes NT1.

Demographics

Since the majority of the epidemiological studies included patients with both NT1 and NT2, there are no valid data related to the prevalence of NT2. Age of onset and sex predominance mirrors that of NT1.

Pathophysiology

The pathophysiology remains unclear:
- It is proposed that some NT2 patients have reduced CSF hypocretin-1 (albeit ≥110 pg/mL), which is low enough to cause EDS but not cataplexy
- Some of these cases may reflect early stages of NT1
- About 45% of patients with NT2 are positive for HLA-DQB1*06:02, which is similar to the general population.

Diagnosis

NT2 diagnosis requires the exclusion of other conditions that can mimic its symptoms and sleep test results. According to ICSD-3 diagnostic criteria, the diagnosis can be made when all of the following criteria are met (➔ Table 14.1, p. 132):

1. Daily periods of irrepressible need to sleep or daytime lapses into sleep, for at least 3 months
2. MSLT shows a MSL ≤8 minutes and ≥2 SOREMPs, (1 SOREMP can be replaced with a REM period within 15 minutes of sleep onset in the preceding PSG)
3. Cataplexy is absent
4. Either CSF hypocretin-1 concentration has not been measured, or concentration is >110 pg/mL or greater than one-third of the mean values obtained in normal subjects with the same assay
5. The hypersomnolence and/or MSLT findings are not better explained by other causes (insufficient sleep, OSA, delayed sleep phase, medication, substance withdrawal).

If a patient diagnosed with NT2 is subsequently found to have CSF hypocretin-1 <110 pg/mL, or develops cataplexy, the diagnosis becomes NT1.

Differential diagnosis

NT2 lacks both exclusive clinical features (e.g. cataplexy for NT1) and bio-chemical markers (e.g. low hypocretin-1 for NT1), and so diagnosis relies on the MSLT findings. It is thus imperative to account for other sleep pathologies that can have similar MSLT findings:

- *Insufficient sleep syndrome*: this is not only very common, but is one of the conditions that can cause multiple SOREMPs on NPSG/MSLT. Actigraphy and/or sleep diary for at least 1 week prior to the MSLT is strongly recommended, and if deemed necessary the sleep studies can be repeated after demonstrated increased sleep opportunity
- *Idiopathic hypersomnia* (➜ Chapter 15): this other hypersomnia of central origin is largely defined by MSLT findings, and like NT2 is a diagnosis of exclusion. Patients to a significant extent are defined as NT2 or idiopathic hypersomnia on the basis of the presence or absence of SOREMPs on the MSLT. However, the MSLT has been shown to have poor test–retest reliability, which may lead patients to be arbitrarily classified in the absence of clear clinical features pointing towards NT2 or idiopathic hypersomnia
- *Other sleep disorders* (e.g. OSA, PLMS, shift work, and other circadian sleep disorders): these can be responsible for EDS and early REM onset on nocturnal PSG/MSLT, but if treated and PSG narcolepsy findings persist, then the diagnosis of NT2 can be made
- *Mental conditions, drug misuse, and chronic fatigue syndrome*: these can present clinically as cases of EDS, but can often (not always) be differentiated by the PSG criteria for NT2

Treatment

The management of NT2 is very similar to NT1, with the obvious exception of not requiring treatment of cataplexy. However, the tricyclic antidepressants and selective serotonin reuptake inhibitor (SSRIs)/serotonin and nor-epinephrine (noradrenaline) reuptake inhibitors (SNRIs) are helpful for the management of other REM phenomena such as sleep paralysis and hypnagogic hallucinations. Sodium oxybate at the current time is not licensed for NT2 in UK, but is used in other countries.

Further reading

Abad VC, Guilleminault C. New developments in the management of narcolepsy. Nat Sci Sleep. 2017;9:39–57.

Drakatos P, Lykouras D, D'Ancona G, et al. Safety and efficacy of long-term use of sodium oxybate for narcolepsy with cataplexy in routine clinical practice. Sleep Med. 2017;35:80–84.

Drakatos P, Suri A, Higgins SE, et al. Sleep stage sequence analysis of sleep onset REM periods in the hypersomnias. J Neurol Neurosurg Psychiatry. 2013;84(2):223–27.

Leschziner G. Narcolepsy: a clinical review. Pract Neurol. 2014;14(5):323–31.

Thakrar C, Patel K, D'Ancona G, et al. Effectiveness and side-effect profile of stimulant therapy as monotherapy and in combination in the central hypersomnias in clinical practice. J Sleep Res. 2018;27(4):e12627.

Other hypersomnias

Guy Leschziner

Idiopathic hypersomnia

Clinical features

Idiopathic hypersomnia (IH) is a rare chronic central nervous system disorder, with some clinical overlap with narcolepsy. Its frequency is difficult to ascertain, but is thought to be approximately ten times less common than narcolepsy. It remains rather poorly defined, and possibly represents a heterogeneous group of disorders with shared clinical features.

Marked EDS is the core clinical feature of IH, but other features include:

- Long sleep duration—typically 10 hours or more for the major sleep period
- Long and unrefreshing daytime naps, usually an hour or more
- Sleep inertia/drunkenness—patients often describe marked difficulty in waking up, from night-time sleep or daytime naps, with cognitive dysfunction, incoordination or confusion, and repeated returns to sleep
- Cognitive dysfunction or 'brain fog' is frequently described even when awake
- Features of autonomic dysfunction such as headache, palpitations, orthostatic intolerance, and cold extremities are common.

Onset may occur at any age but most commonly is seen in adolescence or early adulthood.

Diagnostic criteria

Previously, IH was separated into two diagnostic entities, with or without long sleep time, but this distinction has recently been dropped due to insufficient validation in the ICSD-3. See also ➍ Table 14.1, p. 132.

ICSD-3 diagnostic criteria are:

- Daily periods of irrepressible need to sleep or daytime lapses into sleep, for at least 3 months
- Cataplexy is absent
- The MSLT shows fewer than 2 SOREMPs, or no SOREMPs if the REM latency in the preceding PSG is ≤15 minutes
- The presence of at least one of the following:
  - MSLT shows a MSL of ≤8 minutes
  - Total sleep time per 24 hours is ≥660 minutes on 24-hour PSG monitoring (after correction of sleep deprivation), or by wrist actigraphy plus a sleep diary (averaged over at least 7 days)
- Chronic sleep restriction is ruled out (if necessary, confirmed by at least 1 week of wrist actigraphy)
- The hypersomnolence and/or MSLT findings are not better explained by another sleep disorder, medical/psychiatric disorder, or use of drugs/medications.

Of note, high sleep efficiency (>90%) on the preceding PSG is viewed as a supportive finding for the diagnosis.

Pathophysiology

The pathophysiology of IH is not known. A family history of IH or excessive sleepiness is seen in about one-third of IH patients, suggesting a genetic contribution, but no HLA type or other genetic marker has been definitely identified. Neurochemical studies have not identified consistent abnormalities in monoamines, histamine, or hypocretin in IH. It has been proposed that in some patients, there is an endogenous chemical that potentiates the action of GABA on the GABA$_A$ receptor, and is reversed by flumazenil. Some studies have identified circadian rhythm abnormalities in IH, with a delayed sleep phase.

Differential diagnosis

It cannot be sufficiently stressed that IH is a diagnosis of exclusion. In practice, however, differentiation from other causes of hypersomnolence can be extremely problematic, and sometimes requires an iterative approach, treating alternative possibilities before making the diagnosis of IH.

Major differential diagnoses include:

- *NT2*: there is significant clinical overlap between IH and NT2, with ~25% of IH patients reporting sleep paralysis and hypnagogic hallucinations. At present, these two conditions are largely distinguished by their sleep study findings, although a long sleep duration is more supportive of IH
- *Insufficient sleep syndrome (ISS)/chronic sleep deprivation*: ISS is extremely common, affecting about 20% of the adult population, and can present with clinical features and sleep study findings consistent with IH. It is defined by the ICSD-3 as daily periods of an irrepressible need to sleep or daytime lapses into sleep for 3 months, with a duration of sleep shorter than expected for age, in the absence of an alternative explanation such as sleep disorder, neurological or mental disorder, or the effect of drugs. In theory, the clinical history, sleep diaries, and actigraphy should identify patients with ISS, but if there is any doubt, patients should be reassessed after several weeks of sleep extension of at least 8 hours per night (which should ideally be verified with actigraphy)
- *Psychiatric hypersomnolence*: many psychiatric conditions can be associated with hypersomnolence, particularly major depressive disorder (MDD). Typically, the extreme sleepiness seen in these patients fluctuates more than in IH, but in practice, a degree of judgement is required as to whether the hypersomnolence can be better explained by psychiatric illness. In any case, psychiatric review should be undertaken
- *Medications/drugs*: a complete drug history should be taken, and any sedating medication should be weaned if possible. Patients should be screened carefully for illicit drug use, and a urinary drug screen should be considered during admission for sleep studies.

Other differential diagnoses include:

- *OSA syndrome and upper airway resistance syndrome*: the PSG will identify significant sleep apnoea, but if the predominant picture is one of respiratory effort-related arousals rather than frank hypopnoeas or apnoeas, then confusion can arise. If there is any doubt, a trial of CPAP should be undertaken

- *PLMS*: patients with significant PLMS should have these treated prior to the diagnosis of IH
- *Delayed sleep–wake phase disorder* (➲ Chapter 16): patients with DSPS will have difficulty waking in the morning, but are likely to have a late sleep onset too. There is, however, significant overlap between the two patient cohorts
- *Neurological disorders*: post-traumatic brain injury patients often experience a long sleep time and EDS. Myotonic dystrophy is associated with hypersomnia in about one-third of patients. Parkinson's disease and Parkinson's-plus syndromes are often associated with hypersomnia, and indeed the sleepiness may precede the motor manifestations of these disorders by several years
- *Medical causes* such as post-viral illness, hypothyroidism and iron deficiency. Profound vitamin D deficiency has also anecdotally been reported in some patients to cause hypersomnia
- *Chronic fatigue syndrome*: chronic fatigue syndrome is characterized by chronic persistent physical and mental fatigue that is not relieved by rest of sleep. Although patients sometimes complain of EDS, objective daytime sleepiness is not usually seen and overnight sleep is of poor quality, with a reduced sleep efficiency.

Management

In the context of IH, behavioural treatment is generally not very successful. Extension of sleep opportunity does not usually result in long-term improvement. In contrast to narcolepsy, planned naps are unrefreshing and therefore unhelpful. Non-pharmacological management should be focused on safety advice, particularly surrounding driving. IH results in a significant impact on quality of life, and low mood is a frequent sequel, depression and other affective disorders should be treated.

Pharmacological therapies are largely centred on stimulant drugs, although it should be noted that there are no licensed treatments for IH. Doses of these drugs, including modafinil, methylphenidate, and dexamphetamine, are used at doses similar to those used in narcolepsy. Other stimulants are caffeine and nicotine, with anecdotal reports of transcutaneous nicotine being helpful for sleep inertia/drunkenness. Other approaches to the treatment of sleep drunkenness include the use of night-time modafinil, which for some patients appears to alleviate this symptom without worsening night-time sleep.

However, approximately one-quarter of patients are refractory to treatment with these standard therapies. Anecdotally, a number of novel treatment strategies have been described to be helpful, including $GABA_A$ receptor antagonists or negative modulators such as clarithromycin and flumazenil, the $GABA_B$ receptor agonist sodium oxybate, histamine inverse agonists such as pitolisant, and other non-amphetamine stimulants. However, only clarithromycin has been subject to a randomized controlled trial. This demonstrated an improvement in subjective sleepiness but not in objective psychomotor vigilance, and unfortunately objective sleepiness was not assessed.

Kleine–Levin syndrome (recurrent hypersomnia)

Clinical features

Kleine–Levin syndrome (KLS) is characterized by recurrent episodes of hypersomnia associated with cognitive and/or behavioural changes. It is exceedingly rare, with an estimated prevalence of 1–5 per million, with a male preponderance. Onset is typically in childhood or adolescence, but may occur at any age. KLS resolves in a median of 13–14 years, but may persist for decades.

The hallmark of KLS is the presence of discrete attacks of hypersomnolence, starting abruptly, developing over a few hours. These episodes typically last days or weeks, during which time the patient appears sleepy, confused, apathetic, or in a dream-like state. Sleep duration is prolonged, up to 22 hours per 24-hour period. Patients are very difficult to wake during episodes, although towards the end of bouts they may simply appear to be resting with eyes closed. Episodes recur at intervals of a few weeks to a few months.

Other features include:

- Disturbances of eating—megaphagia, i.e. eating large quantities of food, was previously seen as a core feature of KLS, but not all patients exhibit this, and indeed some report anorexia
- Hypersexuality
- Irritability, aggression, or personality changes
- Anxiety, mood disturbance, and, rarely, psychotic features
- Derealization and depersonalization
- Difficulties in communication or executive functioning
- Autonomic features such as flushing, sweating, temperature dysregulation, or inappropriate tachycardia or bradycardia
- Headache.

A subtype of KLS is menstrual-related hypersomnia, where females experience bouts associated with their periods.

Diagnostic criteria

The diagnosis of KLS requires all criteria of the ICSD-3 to be met:

- At least two recurrent episodes of excessive sleepiness and sleep duration, each persisting for between 2 days and 5 weeks
- Episodes recur usually more than once a year, and at least once every 18 months
- The patient has normal alertness, cognitive function, behaviour, and mood between episodes
- The patient must demonstrate at least one of the following during episodes:
  - Cognitive dysfunction
  - Altered perception
  - Eating disorder (megaphagia or anorexia)
  - Disinhibited behaviour
- The hypersomnolence and related symptoms are not better explained by another sleep/medical/neurological or psychiatric disorder (especially bipolar disorder), or drugs/medications.

Despite the ICSD-3 criteria stipulating that patients are entirely normal between episodes, it is increasingly recognized that sleep, memory, and mood may be affected even when 'asymptomatic'.

Diagnostic testing

There are no diagnostic tests for KLS. The diagnostic work-up is focused on the exclusion of KLS mimics. A sleep study should be undertaken to exclude other sleep disorders. The PSG is usually unremarkable in KLS. An EEG should be performed to rule out epilepsy, and this shows generalized slowing in up to 70% of KLS patients during a bout. Brain imaging should be performed to rule out structural neurological causes, but is normal in KLS (see 'Pathophysiology').

Pathophysiology

As with IH, the pathophysiology of KLS remains a mystery. It is more common in the Ashkenazi Jewish population, and 5% of cases have a family history, implying a genetic contribution. Recently, a genetic variant has been associated with the condition in a whole genome association study.

Reported triggers include infection or fever, leading some to propose an inflammatory or autoimmune mechanism. In some patients, CSF hypocretin-1 levels have been demonstrated to be lower during bouts, although it is unclear whether hypocretin-1 has a causative role.

Standard brain imaging in KLS is normal, but brain single-photon emission computed tomography (SPECT) and positron emission tomography have shown metabolic changes in the thalamus and some cortical areas, both during and in between episodes. However, the specificity of these imaging modalities is insufficient to recommend these as diagnostic tests.

Differential diagnosis

The major differential diagnosis for KLS is psychiatric disease, particularly bipolar disorder. Indeed, there are patients who have been diagnosed with both conditions, and there are hints at a common genetic predisposition. However, in KLS, the psychiatric features will usually manifest and terminate abruptly alongside the excessive sleepiness.

Other differentials include:
- Medications/illicit drug use
- Migraine with brainstem aura
- Temporal lobe epilepsy or absence status
- Bilateral temporal lobe lesions causing Klüver–Bucy syndrome
- Intracranial mass lesions
- Metabolic encephalopathies such as urea cycle defects or mitochondrial disease
- Acute intermittent porphyria
- Lyme disease.

Management

In episodes, no treatment has been consistently shown to be helpful. Stimulants during episodes of hypersomnolence are generally not successful, although management of associated features such as psychiatric symptoms, e.g. anxiety and psychotic symptoms, or headache is important.

Generally, the focus of treatment is prophylaxis, to reduce the frequency and severity of episodes. There is very limited evidence for most agents, although there are anecdotal case reports of patients responding to antiepileptic drugs such as carbamazepine, lamotrigine, and sodium valproate.

The strongest evidence is from an open label study, for lithium, as a prophylactic agent. At target trough levels of 0.8–1.2 mmol/L, treatment with lithium resulted in a significant reduction in episode duration, episode frequency, and intensity. More recently, early intravenous methylprednisolone has been proposed as a treatment during episodes to shorten their duration.

Many patients however are not keen to take regular lithium, and so supportive therapy is extremely important. Rapid diagnosis and liaison with other healthcare and educational professionals is often the most useful approach. Counselling and psychological treatments for patients and families should be considered, to address the impact of this condition on educational outcomes, quality of life, and psychological health.

Further reading

Billiard M, Sonka K. Idiopathic hypersomnia. Sleep Med Rev. 2016;29:23–33.

Lavault S, Golmard JL, Groos E, et al. Kleine–Levin syndrome in 120 patients: differential diagnosis and long episodes. Ann Neurol. 2015;77(3):529–40.

Miglis MG, Guilleminault C. Kleine–Levin syndrome. Curr Neurol Neurosci Rep. 2016;16(6):60.

Pérez-Carbonell L, Leschziner G. Clinical update on central hypersomnias. J Thorac Dis. 2018;10(Suppl 1):S112–23.

Trotti LM. Idiopathic hypersomnia. Sleep Med Clin. 2017;12(3):331–44.

Circadian rhythm sleep–wake disorders

Alexander D. Nesbitt

Introduction

Circadian rhythm sleep–wake disorders (CRSWDs) are an important group of sleep disorders, in which problems arise from aberrant timing of the sleep–wake cycle. When standard societal timetables are superimposed upon this, major problems, such as insomnia, chronic sleep restriction, and EDS may arise. These enduring problems may often have profound impacts on performance, as well as mental and physical health.

Numerous CRSWDs exist. Of these, a very small number are truly 'intrinsic'—that is, due to inherited molecular dysfunction of the pacemaker. Ageing, behaviour, illness, and the environment, may influence many of the disorders, and are likely to have a cumulative effect in any one individual. However, some disorders are more 'extrinsic' than others, such as shift work and jet lag disorder.

Delayed sleep–wake phase disorder

Delayed sleep–wake phase disorder (DSWPD) sufferers have a chronic (>3 months) and major delay (>2–3 hours) in the timing of their sleep–wake cycle relative to desired/required sleep–wake timing. Its prevalence is thought to be 1–10%. It is commoner in teenagers and young adults; childhood onset is possible. Family history is common (up to 40%).

Superimposing societal norms upon this leads to:
- Initiation insomnia and difficulty waking at an acceptable time (potentially resulting in sleep inertia, or sleep drunkenness)
- Chronic sleep restriction
- Excessive daytime (especially morning) sleepiness
- Prolonged 'rebound' sleep on free days.

This all leads to problems with performance across the spectrum.

When allowed to choose their own sleep–wake schedule across many days, patients show improved sleep quality and duration, albeit consistently delayed. There is also a delay in the 'wake maintenance zone' (a 2–3h period of heightened alertness and performance, just before evening melatonin levels start to rise), meaning patients often feel quite productive and alert late at night.

There is an increased risk of substance dependency—hypnotics (alcohol, cannabis, prescription hypnotics) or stimulants (caffeine, amphetamines). Patients may resort to these in an effort to treat their condition.

DSWPD is strongly associated with:
- Mood disorders (major depression, BPAD)
- Anxiety disorders (particularly obsessive–compulsive disorder)
- Neurodevelopmental disorders (particularly attention deficit hyperactivity disorder (ADHD) and autism spectrum disorder (ASD)).

Treatment of these may help improve DSWPD.
Key pathophysiological concepts potentially include:
- Excessive light exposure in the evening hours, potentially worsened by behavioural delays, including habitual (e.g. device use), obsessive–compulsive disorder and ADHD driven (pre-bed checking routines; inability to attend to going to bed); indoor lighting
- Inadequate light exposure in the morning, potentially worsened by prolonged rebound sleep, resulting from chronic sleep restriction; 'clinophilia' (excessive time in bed); lack of outdoor light exposure (e.g. mood disorders)
- Sleep homeostatic function may be weaker.

Assessment of DSWPD

Assessment involves careful history taking, covering sleep behaviours, and including due attention paid to either known or suspected psychiatric comorbidities. Chronotyping questionnaires may be useful; however, they should not replace adequate history taking.

Sleep diaries and wrist actigraphy (for a minimum of 2 weeks; ideally 3 weeks or more if the patient is working or has other regular commitments) should be offered as standard. The mean midpoint of sleep on free days (i.e. sleep episodes preceding days with no commitments) is the most robust phase marker. Additional phase markers, such as measurement of dim light melatonin onset and core body temperature minimum may be helpful in distinguishing true 'circadian' DSWPD from 'secondary'/behavioural DSWPD in some cases, but availability is very limited and needs careful standardization. Repeat sleep diary and actigraphy monitoring is useful for assessing response to treatment.

Ad libitum polysomnography (to patient's preferred timing), is occasionally helpful, as while sleep physiology is normal, the presence of untreated comorbid sleep disorders (such as OSA and PLMD) may hinder treatment attempts of DSWPD. There is no utility in performing MSLT.

Diagnostic caveats include:

- Delayed sleep–wake timing may be 'normal' for an individual
- Parents/partners may have unrealistic expectations
- A 'motivated' DSWPD phenotype has been suggested, in which a return to a more normal function is not desirable
- Sleep inertia, and EDS, should not persist if allowed to sleep for several days at the preferred sleep schedule
- Poor sleep behaviour (stimulus control, sleep hygiene) is not assessed adequately or addressed.

Treatment of DSWPD

Treatment is tailored to the individual. As a chronic disorder, 'relapses' are common, so addressing expectations, and a commitment to treatment compliance, need clear discussion. Some patients may need to accept that profound phase advances might not be achievable.

Behavioural measures include:

- Sleep-timing education (body clock, light, sleep pressure)
- Limiting evening light exposure
- Low indoor lighting levels, ideally floor level
- Sunglasses outdoors on summer evenings
- Use of blue-light blocking glasses (amber lenses)
- Encouraging morning light exposure
- Scheduled (20 minutes plus) outdoor light exposure after waking
- Scheduling daytime activity
- Scheduled exercise, at the same time each day, ideally before late evening
- Scheduled meals, ideally at the same time each day
- Addressing maladaptive sleep behaviours
- Elements of CBT-I, such as stimulus control, setting anchors, and sleep scheduling.

Psychological factors to address include:

- Recognizing and treating/signposting towards treatment of comorbid psychiatric and dependency issues
- Acknowledging interpersonal (parental) dynamics and conflict
- Encouraging ownership of the problem.

More intensive measures, to consider once behavioural measures are in place, include:

- Use of melatonin as a chronobiotic (not a hypnotic):
  - Evidence suggests low doses more effective
  - 0.5 mg immediate-release melatonin = ¼ of a 2.0 mg prolonged-release melatonin tablet, cut with a pill cutter
  - 0.5 mg melatonin taken 10 hours before the calculated mean midpoint of sleep on free days could advance phase by around 90 minutes
  - Should be taken daily at a set time (timed to watch or phone alarm)

- Light exposure (20 minutes), ideally natural, or augmented with a light box, should occur as close as possible to immediately waking, or, if tolerated, 60–90 minutes before habitual wake time:
  - Commercial light boxes deliver 10,000 lux of light at 30–85 cm gaze
  - Overcast sky at midday delivers same amount of light.

If a new, stable pattern of sleep–wake timing is achieved, mean midpoint of sleep on free days can be recalculated, and the treatment timings bought forward again. Typically, up to three serial advances are attempted.

Some practitioners advocate serially delaying patients with extreme phase delays (chronotherapy), and then trying to hold them at a new sleep–wake cycle phase with the above-mentioned measures. This is not widely recommended, unless very carefully calculated and supervised, as it could risk decompensation into non-24-hour sleep–wake rhythm disorder.

Advanced sleep–wake phase disorder

In advanced sleep–wake phase disorder (ASWPD), sufferers have a chronic (>3 months) and major advance (>2–3 hours) in the timing of their sleep–wake cycle relative to desired/required sleep–wake timing. This results in early morning (end) insomnia, and excessive sleepiness in the evening. Chronic sleep restriction may occur if evening activities delay sleep onset. Again, as with DSWPD, when allowed to choose their own sleep–wake schedule across many days, patients show improved sleep quality and duration, albeit consistently advanced.

Prevalence data is difficult to ascertain; it is thought to be <1%, but perhaps is underreported, as it is less problematic than DSWPD. It is more common in older adults.

Autosomal dominant familial forms exist, but are very rare, with mutations in *PER2* and *CSNK1D* genes described.

ASWPD can also be associated with neurodevelopmental disorders (Smith–Magenis syndrome, ASD, chromosomal microdeletions).

Purported pathophysiological mechanisms include the inverse of those relevant to DSWPD, including:

- Excessive light exposure in the early morning, or heightened physiological response to the phase-advancing effects of this
- Inadequate evening light exposure, or poor physiological response to the phase-delaying effects of this
- Clear laboratory evidence from a single elderly patient with familial ASWPD showed a shortened period length of 23.3 hours
- There may be a stronger and earlier drive in sleep homeostatic pressure.

Assessment of ASWPD

Assessment is detailed history taking, supplemented by *at least* 2 weeks of sleep diaries and contemporaneous actigraphy. While abnormally advanced phase markers such as dim light melatonin onset and core body temperature minimum may be present in familial cases, these are less likely to be helpful in patients with sporadic ASWPD, and may not differ from normal chronotypes.

Other than sleep timing, PSG is essentially normal for age, and adds little, bar to exclude additional sleep pathologies, such as OSA as a cause of evening sleepiness and early morning waking (from REM-predominant OSA).

ASWPD needs to be distinguished from 'normal' sleep–wake timing, poor sleep behaviour, such as evening napping (particularly in the elderly), and end insomnia, which can be a prominent feature of major depression. Having lifelong early chronotype sleep–wake timing, in the presence of good sleep behaviours and no contemporaneously emerging mood disorders, can be quite indicative.

Treatment of ASWPD

Treatment is again multimodal, including:
- Behavioural:
  - Regularly scheduled daytime activity
  - Avoidance of evening napping, counteracted with exercise
  - Encourage good sleep behaviours
  - Avoidance of early morning light
  - Evening light exposure
  - Consideration of indoor lighting
- Bright light boxes, when used correctly, are useful here
- Beware concomitant use with photosensitizing drugs in the elderly
- Use of low-dose melatonin (0.5 mg) on waking at final rise time can also be considered.

Non-24-hour sleep–wake rhythm disorder

Non-24-hour sleep–wake rhythm disorder (Non-24) is characterized by a sleep–wake cycle that is desynchronized from the solar cycle. In this disorder, the sleep–wake cycle takes on a period length typically >24 hours, and consequently, sleep onset progressively delays, usually between 20–60+ minutes, day after day.

As such, when patients attempt to sleep at a regular desired time, periods of insomnia and daytime sleepiness alternate with brief, more normal periods of sleep–wake timing, during which the sleep–wake cycle is briefly aligned with the solar (or desired sleep–wake timing) cycle. Occasionally sufferers will delay by longer intervals ('jumps', of up to 4 hours) each day, in an effort to speed up temporary periods of stability.

The disorder can be seen in blind (especially those with no light perception) and sighted individuals. In blind patients, there is disruption of the entrainment pathways, although in certain retinal disorders the melanopsin-containing photosensitive retinal ganglion cells are relatively spared. 50% or more of totally blind individuals may have Non-24, but in sighted individuals, it is extremely rare (prevalence unknown). DSWPD may decompensate to Non-24 in sighted individuals.

As with DSWPD, attempts to self-medicate may lead to drug and alcohol dependency issues.

Non-24 may be associated with other disorders, including:
- Schizophrenia
- Personality disorders
- Bipolar affective disorder
- Neurodevelopmental disorders, such as autistic spectrum disorders
- Traumatic brain injury
- AD
- Optic nerve hypoplasia (often in association with agenesis of the corpus callosum)
- Rett syndrome, Angelman syndrome, Smith–Magenis syndrome (➲ Chapter 22).

Pathophysiological mechanisms underlying Non-24 include:
- The lack of photic entrainment in totally blind individuals enables the pacemaker (and as a result, the sleep–wake cycle) to 'free-run' at its intrinsic period, which is slightly longer than 24 hours ('external desynchrony')
- In sighted individuals, a progressively delaying circadian phase might mean inadequate exposure to correctly timed light exposure to affect a phase advance
- Experimental evidence in sighted individuals with Non-24 also demonstrates significantly longer intrinsic period lengths.

Assessment of Non-24

A careful clinical history, eliciting past psychiatric history, current mental state, and sleep behaviours, as well as assessment for possible ocular and retinal disease is an important part of assessment. Even more so than with other CRSWDs, a prolonged period of actigraphy (at least 3 weeks; ideally a month) is needed to demonstrate Non-24. Melatonin assays, most efficiently those utilizing 48-hour community-collected urinary samples, performed on two or more occasions, ideally 1–2 weeks apart, may show a free-running dim light melatonin onset time, which could be used to make assumptions about an individual's intrinsic free-running circadian period length.

Treatment of Non-24

Treatment can be difficult, and relapses are common.

In totally blind individuals, entrainment can be attempted with properly timed, low doses of melatonin:

- 0.5 mg melatonin (⊃ Treatment of DSWPD, p. 149) should be administered regularly (by phone/watch alarm or reminder) 2 hours before desired bedtime
- This is best initiated when the individual's sleep–wake cycle becomes transiently synchronized with the desired sleep–wake timing as it free-runs
- Alternatively, continuous administration for at least 3 months might be necessary to 'capture' a cycle and entrain it.

In normally sighted individuals, properly timed light exposure is important. They should be encouraged to have very clearly set, and clearly signed light–dark cycles, with:

- Scheduling activity
- Morning outdoor light exposure
- Evening light avoidance
- Nocturnal darkness.

Identification and treatment of comorbid psychiatric issues is also crucial.

Occasionally, short-term and adjunct use of appropriately timed hypnotics/stimulants may be considered; however, this needs active monitoring to avoid dependency.

Novel melatonin analogues, such as tasimelteon, have shown entrainment efficacy in clinical trials of totally blind Non-24 patients, but as yet, no head-to-head trials demonstrating superiority over melatonin have been reported.

Irregular sleep–wake rhythm disorder

In irregular sleep–wake rhythm disorder (ISWRD), individuals lack a clearly defined sleep–wake cycle, and have a disorganized pattern of sleep and wake dispersed throughout the 24-hour period. This fragmentation leads to multiple (usually more than three) arrhythmic, shortened sleep episodes of varying length (usually <4 hours) across the 24-hour period, although total cumulative sleep amounts during this period may be normal for age.

ISWRD usually co-associates with other conditions. It can be seen in:

- Neurodevelopmental disorders, e.g. Smith–Magenis, Angelman, and Williams syndromes
- Autistic spectrum disorders
- Neurodegenerative disorders—AD, parkinsonism, Huntington's disease
- Traumatic brain injury
- Midline brain lesions with hypothalamic–pituitary disruption (tumours, post-surgical lesions, inflammatory conditions)
- Post-central nervous system infection (especially basal meningitis)
- Sequel of whole-brain radiotherapy
- Psychiatric disorders, especially schizophrenia.

It can rarely be associated with chaotic lifestyles, and chaotic household environments are a risk for development of the disorder.

The disorder is likely to be both biological (resulting from disruption of circadian pathways) and environmental (resulting from weak or dampened exposure to daylight and routine—which are more common in institution-alized elderly patients, and younger patients with neurodevelopmental conditions).

Assessment of ISWRD

Assessment can often be difficult, as differentiating sleep from rest in elderly patients might prove challenging on the basis of actigraphy alone, and com-panion or carer corroborative history is invaluable, particularly in patients with communication difficulties. Nevertheless, actigraphy can provide ob-jective patterns which support the diagnosis.

Additional assessments, or investigations, such as neurological referral, MRI scanning, genetic or psychometric testing, or psychiatric evaluation should be strongly considered.

Other causes of sleep fragmentation, or regular napping, including very poor behavioural sleep practices, poor sleeping environments, or comorbid medical conditions should be sought, assessed, and treated.

Treatment of ISWRD

Overall, treatment of the condition remains unsatisfactory, although significant effort should be put into improving time cues, including:

- Structured, and consistently recurring, social and physical activity patterns
- Consistently timed meals
- Prominent time cues (clocks); 'quiet' signs at night
- Separate sleeping and living environments
- Avoidance of prolonged bed rest
- Appropriately scheduled and augmented light–dark cycles
- Augmentation of daylight exposure in care home settings.

Regularly timed administration of low-dose melatonin (➲ Treatment of DSWPD, p. 149) 2 hours before desired bedtime might offer some benefit, particularly in younger patients, although no systematic or high-quality evidence of efficacy exists, and dosing schedules have not been determined.

Shift work disorder

Insomnia and excessive sleepiness result from work hours occurring during usual sleep hours in this disorder. It is more commonly associated with night shift workers, early shift workers, or rotating shifts (where prevalence has been estimated to be as high as 38%) than with late or split-shift patterns. Sleep restriction is often considerable, and sleep achieved 'out of phase' is reported to be of poor quality. In some individuals, these problems may persist for some time after they stop shift working.

There can be considerable occupational health concerns with the disorder, not least in terms of safety (occupational accidents, professional drivers), but also development of additional mental and physical health concerns, including, in some epidemiological studies, reports of higher incidences of metabolic and cardiovascular diseases, as well as reports of higher rates of certain cancers.

Risk factors include:
• Age
• Mental and physical health concerns
• Social pressures following shift work (including childcare commitments)
• Individual chronotype (early chronotypes sleep less during the daytime)
• Individual flexibility of both circadian timekeeping and sleep homeostatic symptoms.

Actigraphy with contemporaneous sleep diaries is again useful to quantify total sleep times across multiple days, and assess daytime sleep fragmentation. Additional sleep disorders in shift workers should be routinely assessed, investigated, and treated where appropriate

Treatment of shift work disorder

Clearly, cessation of shift work is desirable, but not practical in most. As countermeasures, the most useful suggestions include:
• Clockwise shift rotations (normal, late, night, off)
• Avoidance of many successive night shifts
• Where possible, have later change overs rather than very early
• Regular break scheduling
• 2-hour naps prior to starting night shifts better than 2-hour naps during night shifts.

Sleep education among shift workers is also important:
• Encouraging good sleep behaviours and undoing bad habits
• Black out, quiet environment
• Limit interruptions
• Standard stimulus control advice
• Standard scheduling advice
• Recognition of critical times of vulnerability
• If naps needed, encourage shorter naps of 10–20 minutes.

These approaches may be augmented with medications, including:
• Caffeine—used before onset of sleepiness rather than after it
• Consider short courses of modafinil in some cases
• Melatonin (again, using small doses—0.5 mg) can be useful to help facilitate sleep out of phase (daytime).

While nocturnal bright light therapy is also sometimes considered, this should be used with caution, particularly in short-term night shift patterns.

Jet lag disorder

At its most extreme, air crew are at risk of both shift work disorder and jet lag disorder, although most carriers and aviation authorities are proactive in scheduling shifts, destinations, and rest time to try and mitigate these.

Jet lag, resulting from temporary misalignment between the clock and destination solar/sleep–wake cycle, is typically associated with trans-meridian travel across three or more time zones, and is usually more marked with eastward travel, as a phase advance is required, and often harder to achieve than a phase delay when travelling westward. It also takes longer to reset the clock with eastward travel, as 80% of humans have endogenous circadian periods of >24 hours, meaning they are constantly delaying slightly, making it harder to achieve the phase advance needed.

Severity is dependent on time change, and also amount of sleep loss sustained before and during travel, and timing of exposure to light at destination. Interindividual variability in tolerance of circadian misalignment also clearly plays a role.

While it is transient, onset of sleep disturbance, reduced daytime alertness, fatigue, and other somatic symptoms including gastrointestinal complaints, emerge within 1–2 days after travel. This can affect performance in cognitive and physical tasks.

Basic advice to ameliorate jet lag disorder, particularly in patients with comorbid sleep disorders, includes:

- Keeping to origin time on short trips of <3–4 days
- Phase advancing on long-distance eastward trips
- This can be started in advance and should continue at the destination
- Phase delaying on long-distance westward trips (this can be started in advance of travel).

Appropriately timed light exposure/avoidance, +/− timed low-dose (0.5 mg, see ➲ Treatment of DSWPD, p. 149) melatonin use, can be helpful. Note that these need to be adjusted daily to affect phase progressive phase changes.

Short-term use of hypnotics, and/or stimulants, might have a small role in certain patients, but judgement must be exercised.

Various unvalidated apps exist to assist with planning; some use mathematical models based on existing human circadian science (e.g. ℘ http://www.jetlagrooster.com).

Further reading

Auger RR, Burgess HJ, Emens JS, et al. Clinical practice guideline for the treatment of intrinsic circadian rhythm sleep-wake disorders. An update for 2015: an American Academy of Sleep Medicine clinical practice guideline. J Clin Sleep Med. 2015;11(10):1199–236.

Benloucif S, Burgess HJ, Klerman EB, et al. Measuring melatonin in humans. J Clin Sleep Med. 2008;4(1):66–69.

Nesbitt AD, Dijk DJ. Out of synch with society: an update on delayed sleep phase disorder. Curr Opin Pulm Med. 2014;20(6):581–87.

Smith MT, McCrae CS, Cheung J, et al. Use of actigraphy for the evaluation of sleep disorders and circadian rhythm sleep-wake disorders: an American Academy of Sleep Medicine clinical practice guideline. J Clin Sleep Med. 2018;14(7):1231–37.

Wright KP (Ed). Basics of circadian biology and circadian rhythm sleep disorders. Sleep Med Clin. 2009;4(2):99–312.

Jet lag disorder

Further reading

Sleep walking and other NREM parasomnias

Sofia Eriksson

Definition

Parasomnias are undesirable physical events or experiences associated with sleep. Episodes are usually classified according the stage of sleep during or from which they occur. NREM parasomnias occur from deep NREM sleep and often involve complex behaviours that may appear purposeful but are not conscious or under deliberate control. There are a number of different types/presentations of NREM parasomnias.

The most common are:
• Night terrors (pavor nocturnus)
• Sleep walking (somnambulism)
• Confusional arousal.

Less common manifestations include:
• Sexsomnia
• Sleep-related eating disorder.

People often have more than one type of disorder with overlapping features. NREM parasomnia episodes vary greatly in complexity and can range from simple gesturing or walking to complex behaviour requiring high-level planning and motor control such as cooking and driving. There may be violent or aggressive behaviour that might have forensic consequences. Events can last from a few seconds to up to 30 minutes, most commonly a few minutes.

Diagnostic criteria

Diagnostic criteria according to the ICSD-3:
A. Recurrent episodes of incomplete awakening from sleep
B. Inappropriate or absent responsiveness to efforts of others to intervene or redirect the person during the episode
C. Limited (e.g. a single visual scene) or no associated cognition or dream imagery
D. Partial or complete amnesia for the episode
E. The disturbance is not explained more clearly by another sleep disorder, mental disorder, medical condition, medication, or substance use
Criteria A–E must be met.

Pathophysiology

NREM parasomnias have mainly been considered disorders of arousal or incomplete arousals from deep sleep, based on clinical features as well as EEG showing continued slow wave activity, a feature of deep N3 sleep, following arousal. There is a dissociation between sleep and wakefulness during events, based on EEG as well as cerebral blood flow (SPECT) studies during events. Continued slow-wave activity and reduced blood flow has been recorded in frontal areas with awake patterns seen in posterior regions to support the notion of a 'dissociation between mental and motor arousal'. People may hence see and interact, but not be fully aware of their actions, and people are often amnesic for events.

Lately it has been suggested that NREM parasomnias may be due to dysfunction of SWS regulation. People with NREM parasomnias have been found to have a different distribution of SWS overnight compared to people without NREM parasomnias, there are more signs of NREM instability, and the normal increase in SWS and SWS consolidation after sleep deprivation is not seen in patients who sleep walk.

Genetic factors are involved:
- Up to 80% of patients who sleepwalk have at least one affected family member, particularly when symptoms continue into adulthood
- Up to tenfold risk of sleepwalking in first-degree relatives of patients who sleepwalk
- In a twin study, monozygotic twins had a five times higher concordance rate for adult sleepwalking than dizygotic twins
- A locus for sleepwalking has been described in a single family with suggested autosomal dominant inheritance pattern with reduced penetrance.

Epidemiology

- NREM parasomnias are most commonly seen in children and reported in about 20%
- The majority grow out of this parasomnia in their teens but up to 25% continue to have episodes
- Prevalence in adults reported to be ~2–3%
- NREM parasomnias can also start in adulthood.

Clinical features

The clinical features can vary between individuals and may also vary between events for each individual. A common feature is of open eyes and people appear to be awake and can interact with their surroundings. The majority of patients have a number of different types of NREM parasomnia events:

- *Confusional arousal*: the person may just sit up in bed and look around in a confused manner, sometimes appearing frightened, before rapidly returning to sleep. Some events may be longer in duration and can then be associated with more complex behaviours
- *Night terrors (pavor nocturnus)*: the person may sit up in bed, appear extremely frightened, and can cry or scream inconsolably. This is generally associated with an increased autonomic drive (rapid breathing, tachycardia, sweating, dilated pupils, and increased muscle tone). Events are typically described in children, and they are unresponsive to external stimuli during events. The child is usually amnesic for the events, which are often more traumatic for the parent. Events can also occur in adults
- *Sleepwalking (somnambulism)*: the person will get up and walk around and may walk out of the bedroom and occasionally also leave the house. There may be complex behaviour, even though there is reduced responsiveness and tasks are usually performed less well than when awake. There are risks of injury to the sleepwalker as well as their bed partner
- *Sleep sex (sexsomnia)*: this includes masturbation and intercourse in a way that is often unlike the person's sexual behaviour during wakefulness. This can lead to assault or molestation and can have significant forensic consequences
- *Sleep-related eating disorder*: involuntary eating and drinking during arousals from sleep. People may eat excessively resulting in obesity or even eat inedible or toxic substances and may hence be dangerous to the person. Cooking during events may also be dangerous, particularly as judgement during events is affected.

Patients are often said to be amnesic for events. However, some recall of the events or dreamlike mentation is reported in over two-thirds of patients, although this is usually more basic than the complex dreams generally associated with REM sleep. Patients often describe a sense of urgency during the events, and a strong feeling of threat that may lead to protective or violent behaviour that may in turn result in injury.

Some of the clinical features may be due to misperception of external stimuli (visual or auditory), potentially related to the mismatch between, e.g. the visual cortex waking up whereas frontal areas remain asleep.

Events commonly occur in the first part of the night when there is a greater proportion of SWS from which events occur.

Differential diagnoses include nocturnal epileptic seizures (⅏ Chapter 25), RBD (⅏ Chapter 18), panic attacks, and dissociative disorders or confusion due to other conditions (Table 17.1).

Scales and scores have been developed, mainly to distinguish NREM parasomnias from epilepsy, but these are rarely used in clinical practice where the following four clinical characteristics may instead be used to facilitate differential diagnosis.

1. Timing of events during sleep: NREM parasomnias tend to occur in the first third of sleep time unless the person has disrupted sleep architecture. It is unusual for NREM parasomnias to occur in the first 20–30 minutes after sleep onset
2. Number of events per night: NREM parasomnias tend to occur 1–3 times/night, while seizures may occur much more frequently
3. Frequency of events over time: the frequency of NREM parasomnia events usually varies with time. At some points, they may very infrequently, with weeks or months between, while at other times may occur every night
4. Age at onset and development of the disorder over time: NREM parasomnias often start in childhood and many grow out of the disorder in their teens. However, adult onset does not exclude the diagnosis.

The history taking should also include information regarding possible triggers for episodes (e.g. sleep deprivation, stress), alcohol habits, and family history of similar episodes as well as a detailed drug history including recreational and prescribed drugs. The patient should also be asked about signs of other sleep disorders including sleep-related breathing disorder.

Common precipitating factors for NREM parasomnia events include sleep deprivation and stress. Alcohol may also be a precipitating factor in some people. Concomitant sleep disorders such as OSA and PLMS may also contribute by causing arousals from which events may occur, as well as by disrupting sleep and thereby causing sleep deprivation.

Z drugs, in particular zolpidem, have been associated with NREM parasomnia events, particularly if combined with alcohol.

Individual events may be triggered by noise, movement of bed partner, respiratory events, or limb movements.

Recent studies have found an association between sleepwalking and daytime sleepiness, insomnia, and depressive and anxiety symptoms, to support the view that NREM parasomnias are not as benign a condition as previously thought.

Table 17.1 Clinical features discriminating NREM parasomnias and nocturnal epilepsy

Feature	NREM parasomnia	REM sleep behaviour disorder	Epilepsy
Age of onset	Usually in childhood	Later in life, often >50–60 years	Variable, often first or second decade
Timing of events during sleep	Often in first third of the night	Second half of the night	Throughout the night
Frequency of events	1–3 times/night, can vary over time with periods without events mixed with periods with frequent events	1–2 events/night. Usually most or every night	Variable, often in clusters usually with higher frequency of events than parasomnias (1–30/night)
Sleep stage events occur	Deep NREM sleep (N3)	REM sleep	NREM sleep, often in light sleep and transitions between sleep stages
Duration of events	1–30 minutes	Few seconds to 1 minute	10–60 seconds
Onset and offset of events	Sudden onset but usually gradual offset after which the person may remain confused or return to sleep	Sudden onset and offset and often return to sleep unless movements vigorous enough to wake the person	Sudden onset and offset. Often rapid recovery with little confusion
Semiology	Eyes open. Variable complexity, not stereotyped	Eyes closed. Variable, often jerky movements and/or vocalization.	Highly stereotyped, often with dystonic posturing or hypermotor features

Diagnostic testing

Overnight PSG is often used in the diagnosis of NREM parasomnia but the diagnostic value of the test has not been established. The AASM practice parameters advise that PSG is not routinely indicated in cases of typical, uncomplicated, and non-injurious parasomnias when the diagnosis is clearly derived from the history but should be performed when:

- Evaluating patients with sleep behaviours suggestive of unusual or atypical parasomnias
- When nocturnal events are thought to be seizure related
- When the sleep disorder does not respond to conventional therapy.

Typical parasomnia events are often not recorded during inpatient PSG and the investigation is often more useful to assess potential concomitant OSA or PLMS than capturing events.

Management

For most patients, reassurance and advice to avoid potential trigger factors such as sleep deprivation is sufficient to control the symptoms. General sleep hygiene advice should be provided to all patients. If alcohol has been identified as a trigger, avoiding excess alcohol should be part of the treatment.

Medication may be indicated in people with frequent, severe, or violent symptoms. No randomized controlled trials have been performed in NREM parasomnias and there is no licensed treatment. Efficacy data of the most commonly used drugs, clonazepam or antidepressants, come from retrospective case series. Clonazepam is usually used in doses of 0.5–2 mg at night only. Sedation often limits the usage of the medication. The medication should not be used in patients with untreated OSA. Among the antidepressants, a case series showed improvement of parasomnia events with paroxetine (20–40 mg) but in clinical practice, other antidepressants such as clomipramine have also been used.

There are case reports of antidepressants as well as Z drugs triggering NREM parasomnia events and close monitoring of potential side effects is recommended after starting treatment.

Some patients find counselling or other psychological input to reduce stress and anxiety beneficial, but the efficacy has not been shown in the few studies carried out to date.

Treatment of concomitant sleep disorders, such as OSA, is an important factor and studies have shown elimination of all NREM parasomnia events following successful treatment of OSA.

There may be forensic implications of NREM parasomnia events and safety aspects are an important part of management of patients who may get out of bed and/or perform complex tasks. Factors to consider include:
- Ensure that doors and windows are properly locked
- Objects that the person could hurt themselves or others with are not easily accessible
- Wearing nightclothes when sleeping (especially in sexsomnia)
- Consider sleeping in separate room from bed partner.

It should be borne in mind that making a diagnosis of NREM parasomnia is not sufficient for a defence in a forensic setting, as NREM parasomnias are common and their occurrence may be coincidental and it needs to be shown that someone was having a parasomnia event at the time of the act

Conclusion

NREM parasomnias are common. Clinical features can facilitate the differential diagnosis, but PSG may be needed, particularly to assess potential concomitant sleep disorders. Medical treatment is often not indicated, but clonazepam or antidepressants may be used in more severe cases. Randomized controlled trials are needed to clarify the best treatment options. Safety aspects, treating concomitant sleep disorders, and avoiding trigger factors are key aspects of management.

Further reading

Drakatos P, Marples L, Muza R, et al. NREM parasomnias: a treatment approach based upon a retrospective case series of 512 patients. Sleep Med. 2019; 53:181–88.

Lopez R, Jaussent I, Scholz S, et al. Functional impairment in adult sleepwalkers: a case-control study. Sleep. 2013;36(3):345–51.

Zadra A, Desautels A, Petit D, et al. Somnambulism: clinical aspects and pathophysiological hypotheses. Lancet Neurol. 2013;12(3):285–94.

REM sleep behaviour disorder

Laura Pérez-Carbonell and *Guy Leschziner*

Introduction

Rapid eye movement sleep behaviour disorder (RBD) is a parasomnia characterized by abnormal behaviours arising during REM sleep. Described for the first time in humans just over 30 years ago, RBD is a condition of increasing clinical and research interest.

Two forms of RBD have been identified: idiopathic (primary) and symptomatic (secondary). Idiopathic RBD may be the initial form of presentation of a neurodegenerative disorder. The secondary form of RBD is associated with established neurological disorders, such as Parkinson's disease (PD), dementia with Lewy bodies (DLB), multisystem atrophy (MSA), or narcolepsy.

The exact prevalence of idiopathic RBD is unknown, but it has been estimated that it affects <2% of the population aged >60 years. There is a male predominance in the condition, although female cases may be under-recognized.

Clinical features

RBD is characterized by the presence of vigorous movements, unpleasant dreams or dreams of a violent content, and loss of muscle atonia during REM sleep. Typically, the behaviours and vocalizations correlate with dream mentation, leading to the frequent report of these patients seemingly acting out their dreams.

Movements seen in patients with RBD vary widely:

- Range from simple jerks of a limb to highly elaborate or purposeful behaviours
- Since these often involve threatening situations, the movements displayed are commonly of self-defence. These actions may include punching, kicking, or hitting the nightstand. Patients may even fall out of bed. These may lead to injuries to the patient or the bed partner. Bites, bruises, dislocations, and fractures have all been described as a consequence of RBD. Of note, the behaviours while sleeping do not correlate with an increased level of aggression during wakefulness
- Non-aggressive behaviours may also be displayed, such as purposeful movements (e.g. trying to reach something, eating), or clapping
- Vocalizations like talking, swearing, screaming, crying, laughing, whistling, or singing are commonly associated.

Dreams in RBD are perceived as vivid and intense, and their content often includes threatening or frightening situations. In the great majority of patients, there is a recollection of their content. Patients describe settings where they needed to defend themselves from a threat, or being attacked, commonly by an unknown person. Dangerous situations involving animals and sports themes are also frequently reported.

Other features of RBD include:

- Eyes remain closed during episodes
- Getting out of bed is rare, and usually as a result of falling out of bed rather than ambulation
- If awakened, orientation is rapidly recovered
- Events have a sudden onset, last for seconds or minutes, and have variable intensity. Once RBD is established, the episodes may be of nightly frequency
- Since they are arising during REM sleep stage, their occurrence may predominate in the last part of the night.

Notably, many patients with RBD are not conscious of the problem, and there is often a significant delay to presentation. Not infrequently, patients seek medical advice after 10–20 years of disease duration, and sometimes only at the insistence of their partners. The severity of symptoms may play a role in the decision of consulting a physician. RBD may therefore be an underdiagnosed condition, mainly in subjects without a bed partner, or in mild forms of the disease. The presence of a nocturnal witness for a detailed description, and estimation of their onset and frequency, is of importance for the diagnosis and follow-up of these patients.

Diagnostic criteria

Given the long-term implications of RBD diagnosis (❯ The significance of RBD, p. 176), correct identification of the condition is important. The diagnostic criteria from the ICSD-3 for RBD are:

A. Repeated episodes of sleep-related vocalization and/or complex motor behaviours
B. These behaviours are documented by video-polysomnography (vPSG) to occur during REM sleep or, based on clinical history of dream enactment, are presumed to occur during REM sleep
C. PSG recording demonstrates REM sleep without atonia (RWA)
D. The disturbance is not better explained by another sleep disorder, mental disorder, medication, or substance use.

An accurate diagnosis of RBD requires the use of vPSG. During normal REM sleep, muscle atonia may be occasionally interrupted by brief increases of muscle activity, mainly in distal regions of the limbs. In patients with RBD, excessive muscle activity during REM may be remitting (phasic) or sustained (tonic). The total amount of REM sleep and number and latency of REM periods throughout the night, do not seem altered in patients with RBD.

A number of questionnaires have been designed for the diagnosis of RBD. While these may be useful as a screening tool or when performing a vPSG is not possible initially, these questionnaires may result a high proportion of false positives. Hence, in clinical practice, a vPSG should always be performed if available.

The significance of RBD

Idiopathic RBD

The primary form of RBD is defined in the absence of significant cognitive or motor complaints. Although initially, and by definition, idiopathic RBD (IRBD) is not associated with any other neurological condition, it is now widely demonstrated that a high proportion of these patients may develop a neurodegenerative condition over time. Hence, IRBD is increasingly considered an early clinical entity of certain neurodegenerative processes. There is a move to calling this condition *isolated* rather than *idiopathic* RBD as a result.

The most frequent conditions IRBD may precede are PD, DLB, and MSA, all 'synucleinopathies', neurodegenerative disorders characterized by the abnormal aggregates of alpha-synuclein protein in neurons and glial cells.

The risk for conversion increases with time from the diagnosis of IRBD. In fact, the risk for fulfilling the diagnostic criteria of a neurodegenerative condition has been estimated to be at 33% at 5 years, 76% at 10 years, and 91% at 14 years from the diagnosis of IRBD. An overall rate of 6.3% per year has been estimated for the conversion of IRBD to a neurodegenerative syndrome. However, the latent period from estimated IRBD onset until the development of parkinsonism or dementia may last for up to 50 years.

The intimate relationship between IRBD and synucleinopathies is also supported by anatomopathological observations. In postmortem studies, Lewy bodies have been identified in the central nervous system of IRBD subjects; and alpha-synuclein has been detected in skin, colonic, and submandibular gland samples from patients with IRBD.

IRBD patients may show signs and symptoms of synucleinopathies, although without meeting criteria for their formal diagnosis. These include:
- Hyposmia
- Depression or anxiety
- Autonomic dysfunction
- Cognitive alterations (visuospatial, executive, and amnesic dysfunction)
- Subtle motor symptoms (such as hypomimia, hypophonia, reduced arm swinging).

Similarly, findings on transcranial Doppler (substantia nigra hyperechogenicity), abnormal dopamine transporter (DAT)-SPECT, or alterations in cardiac scintigraphy may be found.

Risk factors for conversion to a neurodegenerative condition include:
- Time since IRBD diagnosis
- Older age
- Hyposmia
- Alteration of colour vision
- Subtle motor symptoms
- Impaired neuropsychological tests
- Abnormal DAT-SPECT (with or without hyperechogenicity of substantia nigra)
- Slowing on EEG.

Secondary RBD

The symptomatic form of RBD is defined by the presence of a concomitant neurological condition, usually neurodegenerative, or when RBD onset is attributed to a medication or substance use that may provoke it. Clinical manifestations, both in regard to behaviours and dream content, as well as findings on PSG, are similar to IRBD.

In neurodegenerative conditions:

- RBD is present in ~25–58% of patients with PD, 70–80% of DLB, and 90–100% of MSA
- In ~20% of PD patients, RBD antedates the onset of parkinsonism. A rigid-akinetic motor (over a tremor-dominant) subtype is usually developed in patients with PD and RBD. Characteristically, even in severe PD patients, the bradykinesia disappears during RBD episodes (which suggests a bypass of the basal ganglia)
- About 65% of PD patients are unaware of their dream-enacting behaviours
- This parasomnia may be overlooked or misdiagnosed as confusional awakenings or nocturnal hallucinations in some of these patients, especially if there is cognitive impairment.

Notably, RBD may be seen in younger patients, as part of the clinical features of narcolepsy (mainly with cataplexy, or NT1). Usually in patients with narcolepsy, RBD develops after the hypersomnolence and cataplexy, and is less severe. The prevalence of RBD in patients with narcolepsy has been estimated at 36–43%.

Cases of RBD have also been described associated with autoimmune conditions (anti-LGI1 and anti-NMDA encephalitis), paraneoplastic syndromes (anti-Ma2 encephalitis), and in disorders where brainstem structures controlling atonia during REM affected, such as stroke, or multiple sclerosis. RBD is also part of a recently described entity, anti-IgLON5 disease.

Certain medications can be responsible for RBD onset, namely antidepressants (tricyclic, inhibitors of serotonin reuptake, inhibitors of serotonin and noradrenaline (norepinephrine) reuptake), and beta-blockers (bisoprolol). Their discontinuation may result in the disappearance of RBD; however, it is believed that antidepressants often unmask an underlying latent RBD, and it therefore persists despite withdrawal of the medication.

Pathophysiology

Brainstem structures involved in REM sleep include the nucleus subcoeruleus (pons) and nucleus magnocellularis (medulla). In physiological conditions, the nucleus subcoeruleus inhibits the structures that facilitate NREM sleep. Additionally, the nucleus subcoeruleus may be stimulated by the pedunculopontine nucleus (cholinergic) and the amygdalae (glutamatergic) of the limbic system. The atonia of REM sleep is generated by the inhibition of motor neurons, with GABAergic stimuli coming from the nucleus magnocellularis (which receives glutamatergic activating projections from the nucleus subcoeruleus). Emotional content of dreams may be explained by projections from nucleus subcoeruleus to the amygdalae.

The pathophysiology of RBD is based on the dysfunction of any of these structures or networks connecting them. In conditions like PD, DLB, and MSA, alpha-synuclein deposition in brainstem areas is believed to lead to RBD. In the Braak model of the pathological evolution in PD, Lewy bodies in the medulla and pons appear prior to the involvement of the substantia nigra, in keeping with the clinical picture of RBD, preceding the development of prominent motor symptoms.

In narcolepsy however, the hypocretin deficit is thought to be the underlying cause for RBD. Hypocretinergic neurons have wide projections to nuclei that regulate REM sleep atonia and the emotional content of dreams. The alterations of the connections between the amygdalae and nucleus subcoeruleus would explain the characteristic content of dreams in RBD linked to limbic encephalitis.

In medication-induced RBD, complex neurotransmitter changes in GABAergic, serotoninergic, cholinergic, noradrenergic, or glutamatergic transmission may be involved in the pathophysiology of the episodes. There is no evidence that RBD is caused by dopaminergic deficiency alone.

Differential diagnosis

Several sleep-related conditions may be clinically similar to RBD:

- Abnormal behaviours during sleep are also reported in NREM parasomnias. However, behaviours of patients with RBD are usually confined to bed. Patients with NREM parasomnias are characteristically confused if woken (as opposed to waking during an RBD episode), and usually have their eyes open. In the dreams associated with RBD, the dreamer frequently faces a dangerous situation and fights back, whereas in NREM parasomnias, the dreamer would more commonly run away from the threat
- Prominent motor behaviours and possible vocalizations are exhibited in sleep-related hypermotor epilepsy. The movements in sleep-related hypermotor epilepsy are usually stereotyped and often involve dystonic postures. The clinical context and vPSG (with an extended EEG montage if sleep-related hypermotor epilepsy is suspected) would help the differentiation between these two entities
- RBD-like episodes have also been reported in severe forms of rhythmic movement disorders during sleep
- The presence of confusional awakenings or nocturnal hallucinations in patients with cognitive impairment may also result in a challenging differential
- Nocturnal dissociative episodes usually arise in patients with a past history of abuse, and occur during a clear pattern of EEG wakefulness.

Generally, IRBD should be suspected in individuals >50 years of age, displaying frequent and vigorous behaviours during sleep. As previously indicated, performing a vPSG would be crucial to rule out sleep-related disorders that may mimic RBD, and therefore for an accurate diagnosis of this condition. Of note, several of these conditions may coexist. NREM parasomnias may co-occur with RBD in the so-called parasomnia overlap disorder; and obstructive sleep apnoea and periodic limb movements in sleep may frequently be comorbidities found in RBD patients.

Management

Patients with RBD should be advised to adopt safety measures in the room to avoid RBD-related injuries:

- Move the bedside table away from the bed
- Protect the corners of bedroom furniture
- Consider bed rails
- Have a mattress on the floor next to the bed
- Place the mattress directly on the floor.

Medical treatment may be initiated when there is a risk of injury, if unpleasant dreams are bothersome for the patient, or when abnormal behaviours disturb the bed partner's sleep.

Clonazepam and melatonin are the drugs most widely used for the treatment of RBD, although evidence supporting their efficacy is limited. They have both been demonstrated to decrease the frequency and intensity of RBD episodes in small clinical trials and case series. Dosages of 0.25–2 mg of clonazepam are regularly enough for an adequate response of idiopathic or secondary RBD. Potential side effects, such as dizziness, somnolence, and incontinence, must be taken into account, especially in older patients. Melatonin, usually given at a dose of 3–12 mg, may be equally effective and is usually better tolerated. There is very limited evidence in the beneficial use of dopaminergic agents, acetylcholinesterase inhibitors, zopiclone, benzodiazepines other than clonazepam, or sodium oxybate, and they are therefore not routinely recommended.

Re-evaluation of drugs that may precipitate or worsen RBD (namely antidepressants and beta-blockers) should also be undertaken.

These therapeutic options are symptomatic and aim to treat the RBD episodes. However, these treatments have no impact on any underlying neurodegenerative process.

The management of a patient with IRBD includes deciding how to share information regarding the possible significance of this condition. In the absence of a preventive or disease-modifying therapy, sharing this information may lead to anxiety. However, withholding such information may be considered unethical. Physicians should discuss this matter with each patient and decide what to disclose on a case-by-case basis, depending on the information the patient is willing to receive.

Conclusion

RBD is a form of REM parasomnia characterized by dream-enacting behaviours during sleep. The idiopathic form of the condition is often a prodromal feature of a neurodegenerative process (frequently PD, DLB, or MSA). Secondary forms of RBD are seen in subjects with an already established synucleinopathy, in patients with NT1, as a consequence of certain medications, or in conditions where brainstem structures involved in normal REM sleep are affected. For an accurate diagnosis, a vPSG should always be performed. RBD may be distinguished from other sleep-related conditions by the clinical context and with the findings from a vPSG. The management of RBD includes safety measures and, if required, the use of agents like melatonin or clonazepam.

Further reading

Dauvilliers Y, Schenck CH, Postuma RB, et al. REM sleep behaviour disorder. Nat Rev Dis Primers. 2018;4(1):19.

Högl B, Iranzo A. Rapid eye movement sleep behavior disorder and other rapid eye movement sleep parasomnias. Continuum (Minneap Minn). 2017;23(4, Sleep Neurology):1017–34.

Iranzo A, Santamaria J, Tolosa E. Idiopathic rapid eye movement sleep behaviour disorder: diagnosis, management, and the need for neuroprotective interventions. Lancet Neurol. 2016;15(4):405–19.

Postuma RB, Iranzo A, Hu M, et al. Risk and predictors of dementia and parkinsonism in idiopathic REM sleep behaviour disorder: a multicentre study. Brain. 2019;142(3):744–59.

Schenck CH, Mahowald MW. REM sleep behavior disorder: clinical, developmental, and neuroscience perspectives 16 years after its formal identification in SLEEP. Sleep. 2002;25:120–38.

St Louis EK, Boeve AR, Boeve BF. REM sleep behavior disorder in Parkinson's disease and other synucleinopathies. Mov Disord. 2017;32(5):645–58.

Chapter 19

Other parasomnias

Valentina Gnoni and *Guy Leschziner*

Introduction

The range of unwanted behaviours arising from sleep is wide, and is not limited to the archetypal non-REM parasomnias such as sleepwalking, or RBD. Some parasomnias, such as sleep paralysis and sleep-related hallucinations, are part of the classic tetrad of narcolepsy, but are encountered as isolated phenomena in an extremely high proportion of the otherwise normal population. Others are much less commonly experienced or encountered, but a knowledge of these conditions often permits a rapid diagnosis.

Sleep paralysis

Clinical features

Sleep paralysis is a REM sleep parasomnia, characterized by the inability to voluntarily move the limbs, the head, and the trunk, or to speak, while consciousness is fully preserved. Each episode lasts seconds to minutes and occur at sleep onset or upon awakening from sleep, usually resolving spontaneously. The feeling of being 'paralysed' in one's own body while being fully awake is perceived as an horrific experience which can cause significant distress, and can result in major bedtime anxiety or fear for sleep. A sense of breathlessness is often reported, presumably due to involvement of accessory muscles of respiration. Visual and auditory hallucinations may accompany the episodes. Stress, sleep deprivation, and irregular sleep–wake schedule are precipitating factors.

Epidemiology

Isolated events are commonly reported in the general population, and the estimated lifetime prevalence varies depending on the study population (between 5% and 60%). In one study, almost 8% of the general population and 28% of students reported having had at least one episode of sleep paralysis during their lives. In contrast, frequent recurrent sleep paralysis is less common, and is more commonly seen in patients with other sleep disorders, e.g. in 60% of narcoleptic patients and in patients with anxiety or with psychiatric disorders.

Pathophysiology

Sleep paralysis likely represents a dissociated state with the persistence of REM sleep elements into wakefulness.

Management

In the absence of features suggestive of another sleep disorder, reassurance and sleep hygiene advice should be provided, as sleep deprivation and irregular sleep–wake schedules are predisposing factors. Drug treatment with tricyclic antidepressants or SSRIs may be indicated in persistent cases.

Sleep-related hallucinations

Clinical features

Hallucinations are defined to be false perceptions in the absence of a real external stimulus. Sleep-related hallucinations are described to be vivid experiences typically at the transition between wake and sleep. As for sleep paralysis, they can occur at sleep onset (hypnagogic) or on awakening from sleep (hypnopompic). They can be pleasant, or terrifying, mainly visual phenomena, but they can be auditory, tactile, or kinaesthetic (a hallucination of movement or an out-of-body experience) and they often are described as a strange sensation of feeling a presence in the room, seeing shadows, or hearing voices. Complex nocturnal visual hallucinations are a distinct form of sleep-related hallucinations, which occur following a sudden awakening, taking the form of more complex and vivid images, often distorted in size and shape, and disappearing when the light is turned on.

Epidemiology

Occasional episodes are quite common in the general population, with a prevalence of 25–35% for hypnagogic hallucinations and 7–13% for hypnopompic hallucinations. They are more common in young females. As with sleep paralysis, sleep-related hallucinations can be associated with other sleep disorders, substance abuse, psychiatric diseases, and insufficient sleep. Recurrent sleep-related hallucinations are very common in patients with narcolepsy (33–80%). Complex hallucinations are often associated with other parasomnias or they can be associated with neurological or visual disorders (e.g. Charles Bonnet hallucinations).

Pathophysiology

Sleep-related hallucinations are considered to represent the dream imagery of REM sleep intruding into wakefulness. Complex hallucinations may, however, arise from NREM sleep.

Management

Sleep hygiene measures, and treatment of associated conditions or sleep disorders. Antidepressant drugs may be helpful in carefully selected cases.

Sleep-related rhythmic movement disorder

Clinical features

Sleep-related rhythmic movement disorder (SRRMD), sometimes referred to as *jactatio capitis nocturna* when involving the head, consists of stereotyped, rhythmic, and repetitive movements involving predominantly large axial muscle groups predominantly occurring at sleep onset or drowsiness, lasting from a few seconds up to 15 minutes. The repetitive movements are slow and cease when the subject is disturbed, is awakened, or asked to stop. They are typical in infancy but they have also been described in adulthood. While typically arising from N1 NREM sleep, SRRMD may also arise from other NREM stages, or even rarely in REM sleep. Subjects are usually unaware of the episodes.

The movements of SRRMD are classified into different subtypes within the ICSD-3:

- *Body rocking*: the whole body is rocked while on the hands and knees
- *Head banging*: the head is forcibly moved, sometimes striking an object
- *Head rolling*: the head is moved back and forth laterally, typically while in a supine position
- *Other*: includes body rolling, leg rolling, and leg banging
- *Combined*: involves two or more of the individual types.

Epidemiology

Over 50% of healthy children at 9 months of age exhibit one of the subtypes of SRRMD, which usually resolves in the second or third year of life. When rhythmic movements occur in late childhood or adulthood, they have been reported in subjects with anxiety, intellectual disability, autistic spectrum disorder, ADHD, blindness, and deafness, although may occur in otherwise entirely normal individuals. They have been also described in association with other sleep disorders such as RLS, OSA, RBD, and narcolepsy.

Pathophysiology

SSRMD should be considered a disorder only if there is interference with normal sleep, if there is a daytime impairment, and/or risk of injury. It has been hypothesized that SSRMD may be the expression of a sleep promoting behaviour, a positive conditioning stimulus which facilitates entry into sleep. It has also been postulated that the repetitive movements may promote motor development by stimulation of the vestibular system. Other theories suggest the involvement of an inhibitory mechanism on central motor pattern generators.

Management

Optimization of sleep hygiene and ensuring a safe sleep environment. Tricyclic antidepressants and benzodiazepines may be considered in severe cases.

Sleep-related bruxism

Clinical features

Sleep-related bruxism or nocturnal teeth grinding is a motor phenomenon involving the masticatory muscles, resulting in rhythmic jerks or grinding movements at ~1 Hz frequency, occurring during sleep, and usually present multiple times per night. It can lead to tooth damage and temporomandibular joint dysfunction. It is often associated with morning headaches, abnormal tooth wear, tooth and jaw pain, and can cause sleep fragmentation. Sleep-related bruxism can be primary or secondary, i.e. associated with the use of a variety of medications (antidepressants and antipsychotics) or with other medical neurological and psychiatric disorders. It is often associated with other sleep disorders, such as RBD, somnambulism, and in particular with sleep-related breathing disorder, since the activation of masticatory muscle contraction may represent a post-arousal phenomenon. Anxiety and emotional stress are predisposing factors, as are caffeine, smoking, and heavy alcohol use.

Diagnostic criteria (ICSD-3) include the following:
- The presence of regular or frequent tooth-grinding sounds occurring during sleep, and
- The presence of one or more of the following clinical signs:
  - Abnormal tooth wear consistent with above-listed reports of tooth grinding during sleep
  - Transient morning jaw muscle pain or fatigue, and/or temporal headache, and/or jaw locking upon awakening consistent with above-listed reports of tooth grinding during sleep.

Epidemiology

Prevalence of 14–17% in childhood, 3–8% in adults. A family history is often reported; 20–50% of individuals have another affected family member.

Pathophysiology

It is hypothesized that sleep-related bruxism represents an oromotor response to sleep micro-arousals, with activation of the autonomic nervous system. Different theories speculate on a central dopaminergic dysfunction, and high levels of urinary catecholamines have been found in both adults and children.

Management

Sleep hygiene, oral devices to protect teeth, and stabilization splints; identification of the cause when secondary. There is insufficient evidence on the effectiveness of pharmacotherapy but when persistent and severe, clonazepam, or clonidine can be considered. Other options include amitriptyline, bromocriptine, clonidine, propranolol, levodopa, tryptophan, or botulinum toxin injections.

Hypnic jerks (sleep starts)

Clinical features

Hypnic jerks or sleep starts are sudden, brief contractions of the whole body or involving asynchronically different and isolated body segments. The movements are non-periodic and myoclonic in nature, occurring mainly at sleep onset. They are usually spontaneous but can be triggered by stimuli. The motor activity can be associated with a sensory component, which could be somatic, auditory, or visual; the sensation of falling 'into the void', the feeling of 'shock', flashing lights, loud bangs, vivid imagery, or hallucinations are frequently reported. Sometimes pain, tingling, or a sharp cry may occur. Often a transient autonomic activation can be detected (tachycardia, tachypnoea, sudomotor activity). Purely sensory sleep starts without motor activity have also been described. Hypnic jerks can be triggered by emotional stress, sleep deprivation, nicotine, caffeine, or excessive exercise. They are considered to be a physiological phenomenon of the sleep–wake transition period but, when frequent, repetitive, and intense, they can provoke anxiety and fear of falling asleep, with consequent sleep-onset insomnia and sleep deprivation.

Epidemiology

Hypnic jerks are very common in the general population, with an estimated prevalence of 70%, affecting all ages and both sexes.

Pathophysiology

Uncertain, but probably related to changes in neuronal excitability during wake and sleep transition. It has been postulated that they presumably arise from sudden descending volleys in the brainstem reticular formation activated by the instability of the system at sleep onset. Due to the similarity with the startle response, some authors hypothesize that they could represent secondary motor manifestations involving the reticulospinal tract triggered by abnormalities in the sensory processing. Sleep starts are a prominent symptom in hereditary hyperekplexia.

Differential diagnosis

Propriospinal myoclonus (PSM) at sleep onset, fragmentary myoclonus, PLMS, epileptic myoclonus, or psychogenic myoclonus.

Management

No specific treatment is required apart from avoiding precipitating factors.

Alternating leg muscle activation and hypnagogic foot tremor

Clinical features

These conditions consist of high-frequency leg movements (1–3 Hz) occurring at sleep onset or upon arousal from sleep, disappearing with deep sleep. Hypnagogic foot tremor consists of rhythmic movements of the feet lasting up to 10 seconds while alternating leg muscle activation represents repeated activation of the anterior tibialis in one leg alternating with similar activation in the other leg, lasting up to 30 seconds. They are considered to be benign phenomena. Individuals move the feet and toes rhythmically during wakefulness and light sleep and are usually unaware of the movements. These movements are rarely the cause of sleep disruption, but are often found in patients with sleep-related breathing disorders and periodic limb movements (➲ Chapter 13). Alternating leg muscle activation is also sometimes seen in association with antidepressant drugs.

Epidemiology

Onset in middle age. Found in 33% of healthy sleepers.

Pathophysiology

Poorly understood. It is speculated that alternating leg muscle activation may represent a transient facilitation of a spinal central pattern generator for locomotion.

Differential diagnosis

PLMD, akathisia, tremors, or rhythmic movements of other cause.

Management

In most cases, there is no need for treatment.

Exploding head syndrome

Clinical features

Exploding head syndrome describes a sudden, violent sensation in the head occurring at sleep onset or on awakening during the night. Patients report it resembling a loud bang, a bomb explosion, clash of cymbals, pistol shot, or door slamming, sometimes associated with flashing lights in 10–20% cases. The attacks are usually painless but are certainly terrifying. Attacks last a few seconds and may recur each time the patient attempts to sleep, often causing fear of sleep and sleep-onset insomnia. Exploding head syndrome may present in clusters with multiple times per night per weeks followed by remission for months. The course is benign and it can disappear after a few years. It may exacerbate a comorbid migraine disorder.

Epidemiology

Prevalence is unknown, but is more commonly described in middle-aged females.

Differential diagnosis

Hypnic headache, cluster headache, thunderclap headache typical of sub-arachnoid haemorrhage, or simple partial seizures.

Pathophysiology

Proposed to be a sensory variant of sleep starts, but the neurophysiological mechanism underlying this phenomenon is still under debate.

Management

Reassurance. Tricyclic antidepressants may be beneficial in severe cases.

Propriospinal myoclonus at sleep onset

Clinical features

PSM is a movement disorder consisting of sudden myoclonic jerks appearing in the wake–sleep transition, mainly affecting the abdomen, trunk, and neck. Myoclonic contractions spread rostrally or caudally. PSM at sleep onset is a variant of the PSM seen during the daytime, and often arises in the recumbent position. The jerks disappear upon mental activation and with a stable sleep stage. It often provokes sleep-onset insomnia.

Epidemiology

Few data available. It is a chronic unremitting rare condition with higher prevalence in adult males.

Pathophysiology

Jerks arise from a single myotome and spread rostrally or caudally to the other myotomes via long propriospinal pathways. PSM at sleep onset is usually idiopathic but symptomatic forms are reported in cervical trauma, syringomyelia, myelitis, and multiple sclerosis. There remains considerable debate in the literature about the nature of the majority of cases of PSM, with some authorities viewing most cases as having a functional (non-organic) basis.

Differential diagnosis

Sleep starts/hypnic jerks, epileptic myoclonus, or psychogenic myoclonus.

Management

Improvement has been reported with clonazepam and antiepileptic drugs.

Excessive fragmentary myoclonus

Clinical features

Fragmentary myoclonus is defined by very brief irregular twitches or jerks, in different areas of the body. If visible, they appear as small asynchronous and asymmetrical movements of the fingers, toes, and lips, but may occasionally only be detected on EMG. It can be seen in all sleep stages including relaxed wakefulness. Fragmentary myoclonus is considered to be a physiological phenomenon, and is only considered noteworthy if excessive and disrupting sleep.

Epidemiology

Fragmentary myoclonus is extremely common. It is rarely deemed 'excessive', but excessive fragmentary myoclonus has been found in association with lower oxyhaemoglobin saturation levels, in other sleep disorders and in neurodegenerative disorders.

Differential diagnosis

Physiological twitches in phasic REM sleep, PLMs, or REM sleep without atonia.

Pathophysiology

Unknown.

Management

Fragmentary myoclonus is usually an incidental PSG finding, or is reported by a bed partner, and so almost invariably requires simple reassurance. Rarely, it is symptomatic, representing the only likely cause of sleepiness and an antiepileptic drug or clonazepam may be considered.

Sleep-related painful erections

Clinical features

Sleep-related painful erections are characterized by penile pain that occurs during erections, typically during REM sleep. Patients report awakenings with a partial or full erection associated with deep penile pain. REM sleep fragmentation and deprivation due to the frequent awakenings can lead to anxiety, tension, irritability, and daytime fatigue and insomnia. Typically, no pain is reported during awake erections related to sexual activity. Episodes can be sporadic or can occur every night or more than once per night. Commonly there is no apparent penile pathology but sometimes it can be secondary to Peyronie's disease or phimosis.

Epidemiology

This disorder is considered to be uncommon, and it occurs in <1% of male patients with sexual and erectile problems. It can present at any age.

Pathophysiology

Uncertain. Authors debate the role of the lateral preoptic area, altered autonomic function, or on the presence of a compartment syndrome. Increased serum testosterone levels have been found in some cases. Psychosomatic factors cannot be excluded.

Management

Baclofen and clonazepam. Other proposed options include antidepressants, beta-blockers, clozapine, or tadalafil.

Further reading

Antelmi E, Provini F. Propriospinal myoclonus: the spectrum of clinical and neurophysiological phenotypes. Sleep Med Rev. 2015;22:54–63.

Chervin RD, Consens FB, Kutluay E. Alternating leg muscle activation during sleep and arousals: a new sleep-related motor phenomenon? Mov Disord. 2003;18(5):551–59.

Frauscher B, Gabelia D, Mitterling T, et al. Motor events during healthy sleep: a quantitative polysomnographic study. Sleep. 2014;37(4):763–73.

Frauscher B, Kunz A, Brandauer E, et al. Fragmentary myoclonus in sleep revisited: a polysomnographic study in 62 patients. Sleep Med. 2011;12(4):410–15.

Frese A, Summ O, Evers S. Exploding head syndrome: six new cases and review of the literature. Cephalalgia. 2014;34(10):823–27.

Lavigne GJ, Khoury S, Abe S, et al. Bruxism physiology and pathology: an overview for clinicians. J Oral Rehabil. 2008;35(7):476–94.

Manni R, Terzaghi M. Rhythmic movements during sleep: a physiological and pathological profile. Neurol Sci. 2005;26(Suppl 3):S181–85.

Ohayon MM, Priest RG, Caulet M, et al. Hypnagogic and hypnopompic hallucinations: pathological phenomena? Br J Psychiatry. 1996;169(4):459–67.

Sharpless BA, Barber JP. Lifetime prevalence rates of sleep paralysis: a systematic review. Sleep Med Rev. 2011;15(5):311–15.

Spanos NP, McNulty SA, DuBreuil SC, et al. The frequency and correlates of sleep paralysis in a university sample. J Res Pers 1995;29(3):285–305.

Vetrugno R, Montagna P. Sleep-to-wake transition movement disorders. Sleep Med. 2011;1(Suppl 2):S11–16.

Vreugdenhil S, Weidenaar AC, de Jong IJ, et al. Sleep-related painful erections: a meta-analysis on the pathophysiology and risks and benefits of medical treatments. J Sex Med. 2018;15(1):5–19.

Sleep-related painful erections

Clinical features

Epidemiology

Pathophysiology

Management

Further reading

Insomnia in childhood

Charlie Tyack

Introduction

Various behavioural approaches have been shown to ameliorate sleep in children who have difficulties with initiating sleep and getting back to sleep during the night. The fundamentals of these techniques are the same irrespective of the underlying health or environmental concerns. Essential foundations of good sleep include consistent sleep timings with a nightly pre-bed wind-down routine, which is maintained at weekends and during school/nursery holidays, and age-appropriate bedtimes.

Paediatric sleep changes according to developmental stage. Total sleep requirement tends to decrease over time, but there is significant individual difference, so ideal bed and wake times cannot be derived from chronological age alone. Signs that people are not getting enough sleep include needing over 15 minutes to feel alert after waking, needing to be woken rather than waking spontaneously, falling asleep at inappropriate times, sleeping over 2 hours extra when constraints are removed, and significant mood or behavioural changes after getting more sleep.

This chapter focuses mainly on behavioural interventions to address unhelpful sleep associations that younger children might develop, leading them to 'need' parental presence in order to initiate sleep, and following night wakings. Behavioural interventions depend on caregiver engagement; habit change is effortful for all involved. Central to assessment should be clarifying goals of the child (if possible) and their caregivers. Patients (and their families) and clinicians can hold differing beliefs about ideal sleep, owing to societal, cultural, and familial influences. Beliefs about medications can also play a role: some people would prefer the change be effected via medication than take a more active role in behavioural change. Motivational interviewing can support this process, and SMART (specific, measurable, attainable, reasonable, and time-based) goals should be established.

Behavioural principles

Behavioural principles

Behaviourism asserts that behaviour can be observed and categorized, as well as changed via conditioning. There are two main types of conditioning, both of which relate to sleep:

Classical (Pavlovian) conditioning

- Pairing a previously neutral stimulus (such as a bell or a light) with an unconditioned stimulus that elicits a specific response (like food eliciting salivation), leading to the bell or light (conditioned stimulus) eventually eliciting the response, even in the absence of the unconditioned stimulus
- Conditioned responses can be unlearned (extinguished), e.g. by ringing the bell or lighting the light repeatedly without presenting food
- Classical conditioning is especially pertinent to insomnia and sleep-onset associations.

Operant conditioning

- Behaviour change via reward and punishment, e.g. rewarding a child with a prize for helping to tidy up toys could reinforce future tidying behaviours: the reward reinforces the preferred behaviour
- Behaviours can also be accidentally reinforced, such as if a parent responds to their child when they are misbehaving in the hope of being attended to. Even if the parental response is unpleasant (such as shouting), it may still reinforce the child's behaviour, especially if more benign behaviours are not responded to by caregivers. Thus, shouting might lead to behaviour intensification
- Praise is a powerful reinforcer, so mindfully aiming to recognize and praise desired behaviours while deliberately paying minimal attention to unwanted behaviours tends to be an effective way to shape behaviour:
  - *Positive reinforcement*—rewarding certain behaviours, such as a parent giving a child a tablet computer in the hope of pacifying them if they make too much noise
  - *Negative reinforcement* is the removal of unwanted stimuli following a given behaviour. This could be caregivers reducing their demands if a child refuses to take part in chores with sufficient enthusiasm
  - In both cases, reinforcement increases the probability of the behaviour manifesting again.

The effects of positive and negative reinforcement are influenced by the reliability of the reinforcement pattern:

- *Continuous reinforcement*: where every incidence of a behaviour is met with the same reward, e.g. a parent praising their child every time they do their homework without prompting
- *Intermittent reinforcement*: reward is given but less frequently. This is analogous to fruit machines, which reward gambling sporadically, and are thus highly reinforcing

- Intermittent reinforcement strongly reinforces behaviour, and is especially pertinent in relation to paediatric sleep association issues: parents might strive to maintain consistency in relation to certain unwanted behaviours, but for reasons such as concerns about the child's health condition or their own extreme tiredness might occasionally abandon the agreed response schedule. Occasional deviations from the plan unfortunately serve as powerful reinforcers of the unwanted behaviour, despite the hard work put in by caregivers at other times.

Sleep associations and night wakings

Families with children who do not have sufficient mobility to voluntarily leave their cot/bed often attend sleep clinics for difficulties related to difficulties with sleep onset, and repeated prolonged night wakings, requiring parental presence in order to return to sleep.

Some cultures are more approving of co-sleeping than others: clinicians should therefore explore what caregivers' ideal outcomes look like to ensure that their treatment goals are aligned (see ➋ Chapter 22 for goals of treatment).

Requiring parental presence following night wakings is usually related to the conditions at initial sleep onset (e.g. breastfeeding or massage) being unavailable (Fig. 20.1).

This leads to the child signalling to caregivers, often by crying or screaming at a level sufficient to elicit the hoped-for response (caregivers' responses are also conditioned).

Caregivers find that when they recreate the initial settling conditions, the child may sleep and make it through another sleep cycle, and the sleep-wake-signal cycle can repeat throughout the night, especially after the sleep pressure associated with the first third to half of the night has diminished following deeper sleep stages.

While night wakings are perfectly normal, children with unaddressed health concerns and/or neurological conditions (➋ Chapters 21 and 22) are more prone to discomfort leading to night wakings.

General principles of management include:

- Determining drivers of night wakings, including factors that might compromise sleep (e.g. physical discomfort, health concerns). These should be optimized prior to addressing the associations, to maximize chances of success
- Delineation of bedtime routine, including timings, and the conditions of the initial settling is key. Breaking these down into as much detail as possible, including the differences in approach between caregivers, will help to uncover possible areas for adjustment and optimization

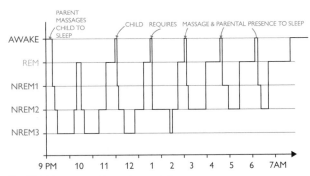

Fig. 20.1 Hypnogram with negative associations.

- Sleep associations can be 'positive' (self-provided) or 'negative' (caregiver must provide)
- Bedtime routine and timing should be as consistent as possible before behavioural interventions begin
- Negotiating how this is to be established is especially crucial in situations where the child sleeps in multiple places, e.g. if they stay at both parents' homes
- Intervention focuses on shifting from the child settling to sleep with negative associations (Fig. 20.1) to only having positive associations—caregiver presence is phased out
- Focus usually first on initial settling conditions, which hopefully generalize to subsequent night wakings
- Night wakings will continue, but the ability to self-soothe means the child no longer disturbs others when they happen
- Transition to self-soothing involves *extinction* of the unwanted conditioned response.

Assessment

Key areas to cover in assessment include:
- Sleep timings, including pre-bed routine
- Family history—structure, health concerns, who lives where
- Sleep environment—single/multiple, bed/cot/other, shared/alone, dark/light, cool/warm, covered/uncovered, quiet/noisy
- Timing of exposure to screen-based media
- Developmental concerns—delayed children might exhibit sleep issues usually associated with chronologically younger children
- Health concerns in child and in family history (➋ see Chapter 22 for more information on 'sleep disruptors')
- Caregiver behavioural management—during daytime as well as night
- Strategies currently employed to manage night wakings
- Sociocultural concerns that might impact sleep quality and environment
- Caregivers' feelings about the balance between approaches that involve shorter episodes of less intense crying, but may take longer to reach intervention goals, and less gradual approaches that can lead to more rapid resolution of difficulties.

Intervention

Various behavioural management strategies can be implemented, depending on the difficulty being addressed and caregiver preferences. The focus here is on strategies to address sleep associations. Regardless of the approach chosen, it is key to re-establish the psychological principles underpinning sleep training methods and explore parental attitudes and feelings in relation to them.

Whilst engaging in sleep training, ahead of the time of initial sleep onset, parents should aim to convey to their child that they love them and are thinking about them even when they are not present. This can be conveyed in different ways depending on their developmental stage.

Sleep-training methods

Pure extinction

- Can elicit rapid resolution to night waking and sleep association issues, though not all families are able to consistently implement it
- Can be used from 1 year of age (if typically developing) onwards, with children who no longer require nocturnal feeds
- Parents often report goals being reached in <1 week with neurotypical children, and sometimes in 2 nights.

The method:
- The child is placed in their cot/bed awake but drowsy, and the caregivers leave
- Caregivers do not respond to the child's cries at bedtime, or during the night, beyond checking that they are safe
- Checking in relation to health concerns may be necessary, and this can be completed via video intercom (if possible) to minimize parental presence
- The child eventually stops crying and develops the ability to go to sleep in the absence of other people
- Pure extinction depends on all caregivers not reinforcing the signalling: if they do occasionally respond to the cries, this can intermittently (and therefore powerfully) reinforce signalling as explained previously, undermining any progress made
- Clear psychoeducation is crucial regarding consistency of reinforcement, as well as the likelihood of an *extinction burst*:
    - Any behaviour being targeted for extinction tends to intensify before eventually decreasing and extinguishing, e.g. children might vomit, and if the parents drop the extinction programme at this point, they might inadvertently train the child to vomit in order to summon them
    - If vomiting or other soiling occurs, caregivers should replace any soiled bedding and child bed-clothing as needed, clean the child up and offer brief comforting and reassurance, before replacing them in the cot/bed awake and resuming according to the programme
    - Historic potentially life-threatening health events the children have been through in the past might evoke particularly strong responses in their caregivers when they signal, making it especially hard for them to resist the urge to respond.

Pure extinction may have been attempted before, but caregivers were unable to resist going in when signalling reached a high intensity during the extinction burst, or if the child exhibited new behaviours, thus reinforcing louder crying or new behaviours. This can also lead to loss of faith in sleep-training approaches. Thus, parents who present at sleep clinics may opt for the approaches subsequently described.

Gradual extinction

Parents who attend sleep clinic often opt for gradual extinction, even though it tends to take longer and still involves crying.

The pure extinction approach is adapted to make it more gradual in two main ways:

Controlled checking

- Caregivers put the child to bed awake but drowsy, then leave
- When the child signals, caregivers initially wait 1 minute, then return, ensure child is safe and say 'it's time to sleep', praise child for staying in bed and leave
- Parents might choose to offer further soothing at this point, but this can reinforce the signalling behaviour so the potential for this to extend the whole process should be made clear during the psychoeducation phase
- If the child signals again, caregivers wait for 2 minutes, and the process repeats as necessary, with duration of caregiver absence increasing to 5 minutes and then continuing to extend by 5-minute increments
- The maximum span is 50 minutes
- Parents might prefer to give reasons for not being present at settling time, like having to check the washing, and leaving for gradually increasing periods of time to run these 'errands'.

Camping out

- Gradual increase of physical distance between child and caregivers, starting with the current settling conditions and taking steps towards the agreed goal—often the infant alone in their cot self-soothing to sleep
- Stages between the current conditions and the goal are established, so that the degree of anxiety provoked at each stage is manageable
- Once the child is able to remain calm at a given stage, the next stage can be trialled, e.g. if a child goes to sleep wrapped around a caregiver, stage one might be the unwrapping of a single arm, then the other, followed by the legs
- Distance from the caregiver at settling is gradually increased until the caregiver is sat in a chair or sleeping on a camp-bed or similar nearby
- Distance gradually increases until caregiver/s reach the door, then move outside the door, then stay outside the closed door
- If a step seems to elicit too much distress, it can be adjusted so that the difference from the previous stage is smaller, hopefully making the anxiety provoked less intense and possible for the child and caregivers to tolerate
- Moving the caregiver out of view can be difficult, and caregivers may need added encouragement and support at this time, as well as forewarning of this possibility
- If necessary, a difficult stage can be combined with controlled checking to help make it more bearable for the child and caregivers. It can take up to a week for the child to become habituated at each stage.

Once initial settling conditions are adjusted to the goal conditions, the child usually adapts to this setup following their night wakings too.

Caregivers should respond in a minimal, almost robotic way at night wakings too, without strong positive or negative emotions being conveyed. This is to minimize the unwanted reinforcement of signalling.

Sleep associations in older children

Typically developing older children are eventually able to introduce the added complication of being able to voluntarily leave the cot/bed.

The aforementioned techniques still apply, but once children are mobile, caregivers need to integrate 'rapid return', systematically turning the child around when they leave their room, and guiding them back to bed as soon as possible with a minimum of fuss:

- Caregivers may describe how their first awareness is waking up to find that the child has already joined them in bed. In this situation, use of a device such as wind chimes triggered by the door of the child's room, a motion sensor, or an intercom can allow caregivers to respond more rapidly, minimizing sleep disturbance
- Elder children might strive to delay bedtime, with requests for more activities like stories or cuddles at bed time. Some caregivers may be more responsive to these requests and some children are more insistent, resulting in the behaviour being reinforced and perpetuating. Thus, clearly elaborating the mechanics of the cycle and the resultant reinforcement loop clear to caregivers is useful. This can be followed by trialling more a more clearly structured approach to bed time
- Reaffirming that a clear wind-down routine is implemented, so that children reach their bedtime having been properly cued into sleepiness is key. Some families might benefit from a clear plan of the wind-down routine being drawn out. This can be in written or visual form, and involving speech and language specialists as needed can support this process.

It is also possible that the bedtime might simply be too early for the child's circadian clock, and caregiver expectations of their sleepiness onset might be inaccurate, as the child's development has altered their sleep timings, or their total sleep requirement might be below average. This can be explored with sleep diaries and/or actigraphy, as well as via clinical interview.

A later sleep-onset time might have also been behaviourally induced, such as by permitting them to repeatedly stay up to wait for a parent who works late to return home, play video games, or use smart devices. In this situation, restructuring the pre-bed routine to make it consistent every night and include wind-down, with at least an hour's screen curfew before the intended sleep time will facilitate sleep.

Once this is established, gradually 'fading' bedtime and wind-down routine earlier by around 5 minutes per night until the bedtime appropriate for the child taking into account their age total sleep requirement is reached, will allow more appropriate sleep timing.

Where children are able to conceptualize and weigh up short-term versus long-term rewards, 'bedtime passes' can be very helpful, and give the child more agency in the process:

- The child is given two or three passes that can be traded during the night with a caregiver for a small reward, like a hug, or small drink
- If the child managed to retain all of their passes until the morning, they earn a better prize the following day
- Provided the right reward for holding on to the passes is chosen, this can be a powerful motivator for some children!

Additional support

Added supports may provide positive sleep associations in the absence of parental presence:

- A cherished toy or an item of clothing with a caregiver's scent on it, can function as 'transitional objects' and make it easier to transition to a settling situation without parental presence
- Aromas of essential oils such as bergamot and lavender introduced to the room at bedtime and removed in the morning
- Constant sound such as white or pink noise played *throughout* the sleep period
- Black-out blinds can be helpful to maintain constant light levels throughout the night, and do not mean that the room has to be pitch-dark
- Dim night-lighting can be employed if necessary, ideally shifted towards the red end of the spectrum as blue light can compromise melatonin levels and promote wakefulness
- If the child has significant fears of the dark, then graded exposure work to address this can help them to reach a point where they are content to settle in darkness, hopefully further supporting sleep
- Some children find the use of devices that light up or change colour depending on whether it is time to be awake or asleep helps to reduce the confusion about when it is time to be awake, and when it is time to be asleep. A readily available form of this is a bedside lamp attached to a timer plug, set to switch on at the desired wakeup time. This can be combined with bedtime passes in order to provide a concrete sense of when the child has reached their wakeup time, and earned the better reward
- Once it is time to be awake, getting out of bed, bright (ideally natural) light exposure for at least 20 minutes as soon as possible in the morning, and preferably some physical activity, will help to entrain the child's circadian clock to the desired wake–sleep timing, as well as building sleep pressure for the next night.

Adolescent insomnia

When young people reach adolescence, the pattern of their insomnia is closer to the adult profile. See ⊃ Chapter 4 for more detail.

The principles for insomnia work with teenagers are similar, with some modifications:

- Sleep onset time shifts around 2 hours later at puberty onset. Some anxious thoughts driving the insomnia might be related to beliefs around their being meant to be asleep earlier than is now physiologically possible. Psychoeducation can address this
- *Sleep restriction* should be to a minimum of 6–7 hours rather than the 5 hours used with adults. This is owing to the longer total sleep time requirement of teenagers
- *Stimulus control* may need creatively thinking about, as often teenagers' only space is their bedrooms. Creating a 'chill-out zone' in their room with a beanbag and some calm activities can be a workable compromise
- Adolescents are more prone to the effects of smart media, so limiting their use, especially in the hour preceding sleep, is key. Teenagers might feel that being singled out is unfair, and it can be helpful to ask the whole family to dock their devices at curfew time!

Further reading

For families

The Children's Sleep Charity. Available at: ℬ https://www.thechildrenssleepcharity.org.uk/
The Sleep Council. Available at: ℬ https://sleepcouncil.org.uk/

For clinicians

Mindell JA, Owens JA. A Clinical Guide to Pediatric Sleep: Diagnosis and Management of Sleep Problems, 3rd ed. Philadelphia, PA: Lippincott Williams & Wilkins; 2015.

Owens J. Insufficient sleep in adolescents and young adults: an update on causes and consequences. Pediatrics. 2014;134(3):e921–32.

Scantlebury A, Mcdaid C, Dawson V, et al. Non-pharmacological interventions for non-respiratory sleep disturbance in children with neurodisabilities: a systematic review. Dev Med Child Neurol. 2018;60(11):1076–92.

Primary sleep problems in the typically developing child

Michael Farquhar

Introduction

Sleep is essential to both physical and mental development and health of the growing child.

In the first 2 years of life, >50% of time is typically spent asleep, dropping to around 40% of total sleep time by adolescence.

During childhood, sleep evolves from the pattern typically seen in newborns, with babies sleeping in 'puddles' of a few hours, to the consolidated sleep pattern of older children and adults. Particularly during the first decade, the underlying architecture of sleep develops and evolves into the pattern typically seen in adults.

Sleep problems in children and young people are common, with ~10% of all parents of children of all ages reporting issues which disrupt the sleep of their child—and their own! While many are behavioural in origin, some have an underlying organic basis.

Conditions affecting sleep quality may not present in an obvious fashion, and formal diagnostic evaluation of sleep should be considered in any child with daytime symptoms potentially secondary to disrupted night-time sleep, such as inattention, behavioural problems, poor concentration, and hyperactivity, as well as daytime somnolence.

Other medical issues which may affect sleep quality are common in childhood, and conditions such as asthma, anxiety, epilepsy, gastro-oesophageal reflux, eczema, constipation, hay fever, and many more, can cause significant sleep disruption. These should be actively considered as part of the diagnostic evaluation and treatment optimized.

A number of conditions which disrupt or impair night-time sleep arise from sleep itself; this chapter considers the principal diagnoses in this area.

Sleep-related breathing disorders

Sleep-related breathing disorders

Sleep is a time of relative vulnerability for breathing, as discussed in ➲ Chapter 7.

Children may present with a number of sleep-related breathing disorders, ranging from the relatively common obstructive sleep apnoea/hypopnoea syndrome (OSAHS) in the typically developing child, to rare genetic conditions such as congenital central hypoventilation syndrome. In addition, sleep-related breathing disorders are found in increased incidence in children with other medical diagnoses, such as Down syndrome, craniofacial disorders, or neuromuscular conditions such as Duchenne muscular dystrophy. Correctly assessing and treating sleep-related breathing disorders in these groups of children can result in significant improvement in both quality of life and long-term outcomes.

Assessment

As in adults, respiratory somnography is the cornerstone of definitive diagnosis.

Children's respiratory and sleep patterns change with age and development, and this is reflected in paediatric-specific scoring criteria for poly somnography:

- Normative data is relatively sparse, particularly in relation to central respiratory events
- It is normal for newborns and infants to have an increased number of central pauses, including periodic breathing, usually associated with a minor degree of oxygen saturation baseline instability
- With maturation of central respiratory control, this usually stabilizes by the age of 1 year. A detailed discussion of CSA in childhood is outside the scope of this handbook; where there are concerns, these should be discussed with a paediatric respiratory or sleep specialist.

The decision to treat should always be made as part of overall clinical evaluation, particularly when poly somnography findings are at the milder end of the abnormal range.

Obstructive sleep-disordered breathing

Obstructive SDB is a complex condition, with an increasingly understood multifactorial pathophysiology, as discussed in ➲ Chapter 7. However, in children with no other medical problems, adenotonsillar hypertrophy is the most common contributing causative factor to significant obstructive sleep-related breathing disorder.

OSAHS is the most common sleep-related breathing disorder in childhood, though there is a range of presentation:

- Obstructive hypoventilation—more commonly seen in the context of other medical conditions such as obesity, or neuromuscular disorders
- Upper airways resistance syndrome—a subtler form of SDB, without the discrete respiratory events seen in OSAHS. However, if this pattern on a sleep study is associated with daytime symptoms suggestive of disrupted sleep, treatment with an upper airway anti-inflammatory medication may be beneficial
- Primary snoring.

There has been an increasing focus on the significance of sleep-related breathing disorders in childhood, as the secondary neurocognitive, cardiovascular, and metabolic consequences of sleep-related breathing disorders are better described. The understanding that sleep disruption in childhood may lead to significantly increased lifetime health consequences means that identifying and treating these conditions early has taken on more importance in recent years.

Symptoms suggestive of obstructive SDB should be positively inquired about, as parents may not always volunteer these unprompted.

Classical symptoms may be present, but significant obstructive SDB can be present in the obvious absence of these. These include:
- Loud snoring
- Witnessed respiratory pauses
- Mouth breathing
- Restless sleep
- Audible gasps, grunts, or sighs.

Parents may also report:
- 'See-saw' (paradoxical) breathing patterns
- Night-time sweating
- Unusual sleeping positions (usually ones which encourage airway opening, such as hyper-extended neck)
- Daytime symptoms, including morning headache, dry mouth on waking, and ENT symptoms, as well as the effect on cognitive functioning and behaviour
- Nocturnal enuresis—secondary enuresis in particular should trigger enquiry of other OSA symptoms.

Footage from parental mobile phones can often be helpful in confirming a clinical diagnosis of OSA.

The disruption to night-time sleep quality caused by obstructive breathing results in fragmented sleep; this in turn can cause an increase in other sleep conditions such as partial arousal (NREM) parasomnias.

Sleep study stratification
A modified version of the AASM criteria for scoring respiratory events is used for children. As well as having adjusted criteria for events themselves, a different severity scale, based on the AHI, is also used.

In children, OSAHS is scored as follows:
- Normal: <1 event/hour
- Borderline: 1–1.5 events/hour
- Mild OSAHS: 1.5–5 events/hour
- Moderate OSAHS: 5–10 events/hour
- Severe OSAHS: >10 events/hour.

Management
In mild OSAHS, or OSAHS with no significant secondary daytime sequelae, medical interventions can be considered in the first instance:
- Medications intended to reduce upper airway inflammation, e.g. montelukast or nasal steroid sprays
- A 'watch and wait' strategy with repeat sleep study at 6–12 months.

For those with moderate or greater severity of OSAHS, or where there are significant daytime symptoms, further intervention should be considered:

- In typically developing children with a clear history of symptomatic OSA, no other risk factors, and with adenotonsillar hypertrophy, no further investigation may be required, and a decision to proceed to operative intervention (adenotonsillectomy) can be made by a paediatric ENT surgeon:
  - Curative in the vast majority (~80%) of typically developing children with symptomatic OSA
  - Generally considered a safe operation, but does carry potential risks and complications, and the decision to operate should be carefully considered. Modern surgical techniques, such as intracapsular ablation surgical approaches, can reduce complication rates
  - Tonsillar tissue does not usually recur, but adenoids, particularly in the younger child, may regrow, leading to a return of symptoms after an interval
- If other risk factors are present (e.g. age, comorbid medical conditions, suspected severe obstruction), oximetry can be used to stratify disease severity. This allows informed decisions about likely need for perioperative support to be made. Children with significant risk factors, or suspected/confirmed severe disease, should be managed in conjunction with a specialist paediatric service, including access to high dependency unit beds
- Children where surgical intervention is not considered appropriate, or where it is attempted and is not effective, may need support with long-term ventilation (➲ Chapter 9). In severe cases, often in the context of coexisting medical conditions, tracheostomy may be appropriate. Assessment and management should be carried out in conjunction with a paediatric respiratory/long-term ventilation specialist multidisciplinary team.

Partial arousal (NREM) parasomnias

During toddler and primary school years, there is a relative increase in the proportion of deep sleep. Normal development of the growing brain during childhood means that children of this age are more vulnerable to the group of conditions under the umbrella of partial arousal (NREM) parasomnia, characterized by states which juxtapose elements of both deep NREM sleep and wake. There is also a genetic element to partial arousal parasomnia susceptibility, and family history will often throw up a parent, aunt, uncle, cousin, or sibling who had similar episodes when younger.

They can cause significant parental concern and disruption to the sleep of the rest of the household, but are usually benign and do not usually result in significant sequelae to the child themself, who usually has no recall of the event. Explanation and reassurance are the doctor's main responsibility. Investigations and medications are usually not directly indicated in children.

Parents and older children often benefit from a 'gear-change' analogy. We shift between sleep stages in a relatively predictable fashion as we sleep each night. These transitions are usually smooth and unremarkable; however, just as occasionally a gear change in a car can result in a missed/slipped gear, occasionally the brain will do the same when moving between sleep stages. This results in a transitional sleep state, between deep sleep and wake, with elements of both arising from a 'confused brain'. With time, the brain identifies and corrects the slipped gear, and returns the brain to a pure sleep stage—either deep sleep or wake.

Sleep terrors

These are more commonly seen in younger (pre-school) children, though can occur at any age. Around 5% of children will have episodes. Frequency generally tends to lessen as children get older.

Episodes can be extremely distressing to family members, and are characterized by:

- A sudden arousal from sleep, appearing extremely upset, frightened, and confused
- Eyes may be wide open, with racing heart, pale face, and clammy skin
- Often shouting non-specific distress phrases, such as 'Help!', 'Stop!', or calling out for a parent/carer
- Attempts to calm or contain the child will often result in hitting out or increased agitation
- Episodes can last up to an hour, with a median time of around 15 minutes
- Episodes will usually burn out, and children will settle back into either normal sleep, or they will rouse to full wakefulness and can then be settled back into sleep. At this point, parents will often need reassuring that they have not just witnessed a demonic possession—the traditional treatment was exorcism—and possibly a stiff drink.

Explanation to parents/carers is often usefully framed around the idea that a sleep terror represents the panicked response of a confused brain, which triggers the type of autonomic and behavioural features usually associated with the 'fight or flight' response.

Sleepwalking

Sleepwalking is more common, with ~20% of children having regular episodes, and ~40% having at least one episode during childhood. It is usually seen in slightly older children than sleep terrors though can occur at any age. Most children grow out of sleepwalking by teenage years; a small minority will persist into adult years (➜ Chapter 17).

Typical features include:

- Events usually occur during the first third of the nocturnal sleep period, when deep sleep predominates
- Episodes last anywhere from 5 minutes to an hour, with a median duration of around 15 minutes
- It is more unusual for episodes to recur within the same night, though not unheard of
- The child may appear in parents' bedrooms, or urinate in unusual places, or successfully navigate stairs, seemingly without problems
- Although eyes may be open, they do not respond meaningfully to direct conversation
- Events will usually self-correct, and the child typically simply needs to be returned to bed where they will usually settle back into 'normal' sleep
- The principal risk in relation to sleepwalking is of secondary injury, caused by the unexpected obstacle in their path
- Children will typically have no recall of the episode the next day, though occasionally some will have a hazy partial recall, particularly of ends of episodes.

Families are usually more distressed or disrupted by the event than the child themselves, and it is unusual for parasomnia events in isolation to lead to significant next-day symptoms of sleep disruption.

Explanations to children and families, in a similar way to that of sleep terrors, can usefully make use of the 'confused brain' idea, with the idea that, in older children, the confused brain rather than triggering a panic-type response instead triggers 'autopilot' behaviours.

Precipitating factors

Episodes of partial arousal parasomnias are more likely to occur in the context of other factors which affect sleep quality:

- Conditions directly associated with sleep itself (e.g. OSAHS, PLMD)
- Other conditions which may affect sleep quality, both physical, such as intercurrent viral illness or full bladder, or mental, such as anxiety—it is not unusual to see an increase in partial arousal parasomnia events around times of transition or upheaval (e.g. return to school)
- Sleep deprivation for any reason will make episodes more likely to occur, as will changes to normal sleep routine or environment (e.g. while on holiday).

Differential diagnosis

The diagnosis is usually clear from the history, but:

- The terms 'sleep terror' and 'nightmare' are often used loosely; however, the clinical distinction is usually clear. Nightmares—arising from REM sleep—are more likely in the latter third of the night's sleep. Children, though often seeming terrified, will be fully conscious, aware, and will give a narrative description of what has occurred in their dreams to scare them
- Occasionally, partial arousal parasomnias may be difficult to differentiate from nocturnal seizures (➔ Chapters 17 and 25). Clinical features suggestive of seizures include:
  - Episodes occur throughout the sleep period
  - Significant daytime symptoms (particularly next-day sleepiness) not explicable by other causes
  - Multiple episodes regularly occur within single nights
  - Enuresis may occur in association with partial arousal episodes (and can be relatively common in its own right), but regular nocturnal enuresis in association with night-time episodes should prompt consideration of seizures.

Investigations

The diagnosis can usually be confidently made from the history, but in certain situations investigations may be warranted:

- Where there is a clinical suspicion that conditions such as OSAHS or PLMD may be present and contributing to sleep fragmentation and acting as triggers, PSG may be indicated
- Video recording of episodes on parental mobile phones may aid diagnosis; this can be particularly helpful where seizures are suspected
- Definitive diagnosis of nocturnal seizures can be challenging, and may require combined vPSG/EEG telemetry—this then depends on an episode occurring during the investigation period. Repeat investigation may be required.

Management

Confident explanation, reassurance, and advice regarding conservative measures are paramount:

- Good core sleep routine and habits should be strongly encouraged
- For sleepwalking, strategies should be put in place to minimize risk of harm. Doors and windows should be securely locked. A bell tied to the back of the child's bedroom door can alert parents to children's nocturnal peregrination
- There is no benefit to waking a child during an event. While this will not, as the old wives' tales cautioned, result in death, it will result in an awake, confused child with no benefit. Children woken from a sleep terror will experience all the visceral symptoms of pure fear, with no understanding for why they feel like this. Simply guiding the child back to bed is all that is usually required. There is equally little benefit in discussing night-time events with the child the next day

- If events occur regularly and frequently at a predictable time, then scheduled awakening—lightly waking the child—about 15–20 minutes before the expected time of the event for a period of 2–4 weeks can help to break the cycle in some children.

Specific medical interventions:
- Other conditions contributing to sleep disruption, e.g. OSA and PLMD, should be evaluated and treated where present
- Medication is very rarely required, and should only be considered where events are frequent and/or severe, resulting in significant risk of harm to the child or of disruption to the family. Rapid-acting benzodiazepines and tricyclic antidepressants can be used, though this should be in discussion with a paediatric sleep specialist.

Movements in sleep

Movements in sleep are likely to be normal, but abnormal movements in sleep can be seen in a number of conditions. These include any conditions which disrupt sleep quality, with movements been seen in conjunction with the arousals which result.

Restless legs syndrome/periodic limb movement disorder

These conditions, discussed in more detail in ➡ Chapter 13, are also relatively common in children and young people, with an estimated probable prevalence of ~5%. They are almost certainly significantly underdiagnosed in children and young people.

Diagnosis of RLS can be less clear cut in children, especially younger children, who may describe the classical sensory symptoms of RLS in much more general terms of 'aches and pains'. This can often be put down to 'growing pains'.

A typical history consists of:
• Described or apparent leg discomfort, relieved by movement, especially in the evening or at night
• A history of delayed sleep onset
• A family history can be helpful—and it is not unusual to diagnose both parent and child in the paediatric clinic!
• Open-ended questioning about 'funny feelings' in limbs at sleep onset may be rewarded with descriptive terms such as 'my legs feel fizzy' or 'it feels like invisible creepy-crawlies'.

Additional features may include:
• PLMS, with a history of significant night-time fidgeting, 'kicking' in sleep, or generally increased body movements in sleep. PLMS may be isolated, i.e. in the absence of RLS, which requires PSG for diagnosis
• Daytime symptoms of inattention, hyperactivity, or poor concentration (as with any condition affecting sleep quality).
• RLS symptoms and PLMS are more often found in children with diagnoses of narcolepsy and ADHD, among others. There is a high association of PLMS with OSA.

Treatment focuses primarily on:
• Optimizing core sleep routine and habits
• Avoidance of substances likely to worsen RLS/PLMD, e.g. caffeine or medications, including sedative antihistamines, sometimes prescribed to aid sleep difficulties in children
• Non-pharmacological strategies such as exercise a few hours before bedtime
• Maintenance of adequate iron levels (➡ Chapter 13). Although most paediatric reference laboratories will report a ferritin level of ~30 micrograms/L as 'normal', if there is a possible diagnosis of RLS/PLMD, empirical trial of oral iron supplementation if ferritin is <50 micrograms/L should be considered, aiming for a target of 50–80 micrograms/L in the first instance. For children and young people with clear RLS/PLMD, and ferritin <30 micrograms/L, intravenous iron infusion can result in rapid resolution of symptoms
• If additional drug treatments are felt to be indicated for children with RLS/PLMD, this should always be discussed with a paediatric sleep specialist with experience in treating these conditions.

Rhythmic movement disorders of sleep

These are relatively common, usually benign, and are more likely to cause concern to families than to children themselves.

They are characterized by:

- Repetitive, rhythmic, stereotyped movements of large muscle groups, typically headbanging or body rocking/rolling. They are most commonly self-soothing behaviours (analogous to thumb sucking) and are typically seen at sleep onset
- Can be accompanied by rhythmic noises (e.g. humming)
- Can also be present during daytime periods of relative inattention (e.g. watching television) or when stressed or upset
- May recur at intervals throughout the night, in association with the normal pattern of arousal and settling back into sleep
- Any condition which increases sleep disruption may result in increased frequency of rhythmic movements.

Other key features:

- Common: ~60% of infants <1year, 33% of 18-month-olds, 5% of 5-year-olds
- Usually reduce in frequency with age
- Although more common in children with neurodevelopmental disorders, most children who engage in these behaviours are developmentally normal
- Can be distracted out of them; parental attention often reinforces rather than reduces frequency.

The main source of concern is from parents, who may be worried that children will injure themselves (this is relatively rare), or due to disruption to the rest of the family from noise associated with the movements.

Management

- Reassurance and explanation
- Protective measures (e.g. cot bumpers or helmets) are not needed
- Ensure bed is safe (movements may loosen screws)
- Minimize attention paid/reinforcement from parental attention
- Reduce secondary noise—move beds away from walls
- Optimize core sleep routine/habits (for younger children, increasing sleep time (daytime naps, earlier bedtime) may reduce frequency)
- Identify and treat any other factors which may be affecting sleep quality
- Consider use of a hammock.

Additional management strategies, including medication or sleep restriction, are rarely needed, and should be considered only in discussion with a paediatric sleep specialist.

Bruxism (teeth grinding)

(See also ➲ Chapter 19)

- Common (~15% of all children)
- More common in those with anxiety, but most childhood teeth-grinders do not have an anxiety disorder
- Annoying but not harmful
- If occurring regularly, should be reviewed by a dentist 6-monthly—a small minority may benefit from a nocturnal mouth guard to reduce secondary dental abrasion
- Optimize core sleep routine and habits.

Hypersomnias

Hypersomnia, principally manifesting as EDS, is unusual in prepubertal children. Daytime sleepiness in children of this age should be considered pathological until proven otherwise. It is usually the consequence of either a primary sleep disorder (e.g. OSA or narcolepsy), or the secondary result of other factors which may affect sleep quality.

Daytime sleepiness in adolescents can often present more of a challenge. Biological changes in the natural timing of sleep, combined with social pressures which make achieving the required sleep duration more problematic, mean that teenagers are much more likely to be sleepy in the daytime.

Thorough evaluation of the sleepy teenager, considering all possible causes, is therefore essential.

Narcolepsy

Narcolepsy, discussed in more detail in ➋ Chapter 14, commonly develops during childhood, particularly during teenage years. A small minority may present in prepubertal years, and it can present in toddlers.

Successful diagnosis and management of narcolepsy in children and young people requires a high index of suspicion, close communication with families and schools, and involvement of a multidisciplinary team with experience in managing narcolepsy.

A significant number of patients who develop narcolepsy during childhood and adolescence do not have their symptoms correctly recognized for many years after symptom onset. Delayed diagnosis contributes significantly to secondary problems, including mental health issues such as depression and anxiety, which are often seen in adult patients. Delayed diagnosis also results in suboptimal educational achievement for children and young people with narcolepsy, again with significant potential secondary consequence.

Narcolepsy is probably as prevalent in the paediatric population as genetic disorders such as cystic fibrosis. It occurs equally often in boys and girls.

The Pandemrix® swine influenza vaccine was associated with an increase in cases of narcolepsy, including in children and adolescents, in 2009–2010. It remains unclear whether Pandemrix® caused narcolepsy in these cases, or whether it triggered narcolepsy symptoms to develop in individuals who were already at increased risk of developing narcolepsy in their lifetime. Of note, there was also an increase in reported cases of narcolepsy in China, where Pandemrix® was not used, in response to swine influenza itself.

The increased public attention and awareness of narcolepsy symptoms, particularly in children and young people, has also meant that young people with narcolepsy symptoms who had not had Pandemrix® were more likely than before to be referred for specialist assessment.

Presentation

Cardinal symptoms of narcolepsy are the same in childhood as in adults, but may be relatively obscured. Historically, childhood presentations have resulted in misdiagnoses of a range of conditions including epilepsy, psychiatric disorders, and faints.

- EDS—in primary school-age children, this should be considered pathological until proven otherwise

- Cataplexy (may not be present at symptom onset):
  - If present, is usually diagnostic
  - Relatively few conditions mimic cataplexy, including Niemann–Pick disease type C, structural brain lesions, and Prader–Willi syndrome
  - In younger patients particularly, may present in an atypical fashion at disease onset, with 'cataplectic facies'. This results in more prolonged episodes of cataplexy affecting facial muscles particularly, leading to grimacing, tongue thrusting, or tic-like movements which may worsen with emotional stimulus. This can lead to misdiagnosis of dystonia, complex movement disorder, or tic disorder
- Hypnagogic/hypnopompic hallucinations and sleep paralysis. Although commonly seen in patients with narcolepsy, children may have difficulty in describing these phenomena. A high index of suspicion must be maintained when children report distressing night-time occurrences
- Nocturnal sleep disruption
- Automatic behaviours and microsleeps—in children, these can result in apparent semi-directed behaviours, often with repetitive activities. They may be mistaken for daydreaming, absences, or complex partial seizures.

In addition:
- Increased incidence of other sleep disorders, including OSA, PLMD, and partial arousal parasomnias. Where possible, these should be identified and treated concurrently
- Often concurrent significant weight gain over the same time period daytime sleepiness develops
- Precocious puberty is more common.

Diagnosis

Adult criteria form the basis for paediatric diagnosis (for further details, see ➲ Chapter 14), but need to be considered in the context of the child's age and developmental stage:
- In adults, the MSLT is considered invalid if <6 hours of sleep have been obtained prior to it. In children and adolescents, who have greater physiological need for sleep, sleepiness secondary to insufficient sleep may result in a seemingly positive MSLT. Conversely, longer MSLs (10–15 minutes rather than ≤8 minutes) may be seen in children with narcolepsy on MSLT
- Diagnostic evaluation of children presenting with possible narcolepsy should be carried out by paediatric sleep specialists, in a sleep laboratory with sufficient experience in carrying these out in children, particularly MSLT
- Actigraphy prior to MSLT is essential to allow proper evaluation of sleep duration, pattern, and to provide baseline information on sleep quality
- On MSLT, REM sleep more often arises from N1 sleep in narcolepsy, whereas REM arising from N2 sleep is more often seen in the context of insufficient sleep
- HLA testing may be helpful, but is not diagnostic

- CSF hypocretin-1 assay has high sensitivity/specificity in those with cataplexy, but is rarely needed as part of paediatric diagnostic work-up. It may be helpful when symptoms are not clear-cut, and MSLT is difficult to interpret
- Neuroimaging is not essential but should be considered if there is sudden onset of symptoms, if there are neurological abnormalities on examination, or if there is a history of head injury before symptom onset.

Management

The management of children with narcolepsy must be carried out in partnership with a paediatric sleep multidisciplinary team. The aim is to improve control of symptoms; a cure is not possible. A holistic approach is essential, incorporating:

- Non-pharmacological treatments:
  - Patient and family education about narcolepsy
  - Establishment and reinforcement of core sleep routine and habits, with an emphasis on optimizing night-time sleep quality as much as possible
  - Scheduled short naps (10–20 minutes)
  - Weight management
- Pharmacological treatments:
  - Daytime stimulants:
    - Methylphenidate (typically extended release)
    - Modafinil
  - Anticataplectic agents (e.g. venlafaxine)
  - Drugs treating both EDS and cataplexy (e.g. sodium oxybate and pitolisant)
- Educational support—teachers must have good understanding of the symptoms of narcolepsy and how these may present during school hours:
  - Understanding microsleeps and automatic behaviours is essential
  - Simple strategies (e.g. classroom seating position)
  - Incorporation of regular naps as required
  - Specific support around exams.

With early diagnosis and establishment of treatment, it is often possible to significantly normalize quality of life for young people with a diagnosis of narcolepsy. Children and young people should be supported to take part in normal activities as much as possible, with some modifications, e.g. appropriate supervision during activities such as swimming for those with cataplexy.

Medication strategies aim to reduce daytime sleepiness in the first instance:

- Methylphenidate remains the first choice, due to greater experience and knowledge of using this in children and young people. Although not a direct treatment for either nocturnal sleep disturbance or cataplexy, these symptoms often improve as daytime sleepiness abates
- Cataplexy medication should usually only be started only if symptoms are disruptive to normal activities, or if fear of cataplexy leads to avoidance of situations likely to trigger an event

- Prescription of sodium oxybate (Xyrem®) for narcolepsy in the UK is strictly limited to centres specializing in assessment and management of paediatric narcolepsy only. It can currently only be prescribed in postpubertal young people with narcolepsy with cataplexy, where all other treatment strategies have been unsuccessful in achieving adequate symptom control.

Idiopathic hypersomnia

Idiopathic hypersomnia, discussed in more detail in Chapter 16, can present in adolescents, though is rarely seen in younger children. It can sometimes be triggered by other illnesses (e.g. Guillain–Barré syndrome or Epstein-Barr Virus), or following head injury.

Evaluation requires a thorough history, examination, and appropriate investigations, and should be discussed with a paediatric sleep specialist.

Kleine–Levin syndrome

KLS is an exceedingly rare condition, and is discussed in more detail in ➲ Chapter 15.

Its age of onset is often in adolescence, and it is important that those evaluating teenagers with hypersomnolence presentations are aware of it.

Where a KLS diagnosis is being considered, this should always be discussed with a paediatric sleep specialist.

Circadian rhythm disorders

Recognizing circadian rhythm disorders in children and young people needs a good understanding of the normal changes in sleep–wake timing and pattern which occurs from birth to adolescence. Detailed evaluation of circadian rhythm disorders in childhood often benefits from the use of actigraphy over a 2–4-week period, to objectively demonstrate patterns of sleep timing.

The most common circadian rhythm sleep–wake disorder presenting during childhood and adolescence is delayed sleep–wake phase disorder.

Other circadian rhythm disorders in childhood, including advanced sleep–wake phase disorder or non-24-hour sleep–wake phase disorder, are less common; these conditions are discussed in more detail in ➌ Chapter 16. Their assessment and management in children and young people should always involve a paediatric sleep specialist.

Treatment of circadian rhythm disorders can be challenging, and usually requires a high degree of motivation and understanding on the part of the patient and their family.

Adolescent sleep and delayed sleep–wake phase disorder

There is a normal shift in timing of sleep as children enter puberty; for most this results in a delay in sleep onset of 1–2 hours. This results in a physiological sleep onset time for many teenagers of between 10 pm and midnight.

There is a wide range in normal sleep requirement times in adolescents, of between 7 and 11 hours. The typical median sleep requirement time for teenagers is around 9.5 hours. Social requirements—principally attending school—mean that many teenagers struggle to fit in the correct amount of sleep that they need. A teenager with a physiological sleep onset time of midnight, and a 9.5-hour sleep requirement time, who needs to get up at 7 am to go to school each morning will be sleep deprived by 2.5 hours every night. Chronic sleep deprivation is common among adolescents. It can contribute to physical and mental health difficulties, affect academic performance at school, and adversely affect symptom control of other medical problems such as diabetes or epilepsy.

For some teenagers, the circadian clock shifts even further, resulting in a persistent sleep onset time of after midnight. This can then result in significant daytime symptoms, including daytime sleepiness which may be mistaken for a hypersomnolence presentation, as well as mood, behaviour, and cognitive sequelae.

Comprehensive evaluation is required. Treatment rests on educating teenagers, families, and teachers about 'normal' adolescent sleep, and emphasizing the importance of good core sleep routine s and habits. Motivation is key. Crucially, sleep routines must make physiological sense—setting a sleep time which is too early for a teenager's individual body clock will simply result in increased anxiety and frustration around bedtime, which often exacerbates problems.

The effects of screen devices/electronic light on sleep phase should be clearly explained, and the reasons for recommending an electronic curfew from no later than 10 pm each night given such that teenagers understand why this is important.

A consistent wake time, including at weekends, with exposure to bright, preferably natural, light as early in the day as possible, helps to encourage earlier shifting of the circadian clock. This can be supported through appropriate use of melatonin to encourage consistent sleep onset, and—particularly in winter—the use of early morning bright light lamps.

For teenagers whose body clock has shifted such that physiological sleep onset time is significantly delayed (by several hours), chronotherapy strategies, where the wake/sleep timing is shifted forward over a 7–10-day period can be effective. This should be done in consultation with a paediatric sleep specialist.

Further reading

For patients/families

Dawson J, Hewitt O. Mind Your Head. London: Hot Key Books. [An excellent guide for young adults on mental health issues in adolescence in general.]

NHS Choices. Children's Sleep. Available at: ℘ https://www.nhs.uk/live-well/sleep-and-tiredness/healthy-sleep-tips-for-children/

NHS Choices. Teenager's Sleep. Available at: ℘ https://www.nhs.uk/live-well/sleep-and-tiredness/sleep-tips-for-teenagers/

Raising Children Network. Available at: ℘ "http://raisingchildren.net.au/" http://raisingchildren.net.au/

For clinicians

Kaditis AG, Alonso Alvarez ML, Boudewyns A, et al. Obstructive sleep disordered breathing in 2- to 18 year-old children: diagnosis and management. Eur Respir J. 2016;47(1):69–94.

Mindell JA, Owen J. A Clinical Guide to Pediatric Sleep: Diagnosis and Management of Sleep Problems, 3rd ed. Philadelphia, PA: Lippincott Williams & Wilkins; 2015.

Turnbull JR, Farquhar M. Fifteen-minute consultation on problems in the healthy child: sleep. Arch Dis Child Educ Pract Ed. 2016;101(4):175–80.

Paediatric neurodisability and sleep

Paul Gringras

Introduction

Neurodisability is an umbrella term for conditions associated with impairment involving the nervous system and includes conditions such as autism, cerebral palsy, and epilepsy; it is not uncommon for such conditions to co-occur. Rates of neurodisability are estimated as 8.8% of boys and 5.8% of girls. Many of these children and young people have difficulties in many areas of daily living and reports have highlighted the inequalities and poor standards of care experienced by such individuals with learning disabilities in the UK.

Paediatric sleep disorders are easily missed; instead of simply being sleepy during the day, children who have slept poorly are more likely to present as irritable and hyperactive, with poorer memory and impaired learning. Such difficulties in recognition are further compounded in children with neurodisability who may have limited communication skills, yet sleep difficulties disproportionately affect this group of children.

Sleep problems in these vulnerable populations begin at a young age, tend to persist, and are detrimental to the physical and mental health of the children and their caregivers.

This chapter is focused on the management of what is usually classed broadly as insomnia in association with neurodisability. This includes problems with sleep associations, sleep onset, and sleep maintenance with associated daytime impairments.

This chapter summarizes general issues relevant for this population, but also focuses on some specific neurodisabilities, their particular associated sleep problems, and their management.

This chapter is not focused on the management of all the specific sleep disorders that can co-occur in paediatric neurodisability, as in general they should be managed as described in previous chapters on paediatric sleep problems.

Goals of treatment

A failure to clearly agree defined treatment targets has impeded interpretation of much paediatric neurodisability research, and can also hinder effective clinical management.

The outcomes of a sleep intervention desired by carers is often different to that desired by the child, and different again to those intended by clinicians or researchers. A successful intervention needs to define realistic agreed outcomes that can be systematically monitored.

Subjective sleep outcomes

Child related

These usually rely on the use of parent proxy standardized questionnaires. While the 'ideal' questionnaire may still need designing, those used commonly clinically and for research include:

- The Children's Sleep Habits Questionnaire (CSHQ)
- The Sleep Disturbance Scale for Children (SDSC)
- The Composite Sleep Disorder Index (CSDI).

Parent/carer related

Capturing the impact of the child's sleep on their parents and carers is equally important. Caring for a child with severe sleep difficulties impacts mental health, divorce rates, and employment.

Two recent trials of melatonin for children with autism and neurodisability showed that after successful treatment of the children's sleep problems there was a reduction in the parents' daytime sleepiness (as measured by the Epworth Sleepiness Scale) and an improvement in parents quality of life as measured by the WHO-5.

Objective sleep outcomes

- The sleep diary. Whether paper based or electronic, this is still the most reliable. The limitations are obvious and exhausted parents can easily overestimate sleep latency and underestimate night wakings
- Actigraphy has a growing acceptance and provides a more objective measure than parent report, and has gained popularity due to its ability to measure sleep–wake patterns for extended periods of time in the child's natural environment. Studies are using actigraphy in parents/carers to allow a more objective understanding of the impact of children's sleep on their caregivers. This strategy is arguably powerful when the child is also wearing an actiwatch allowing comparison, and a better understanding of mechanisms and impact of sleep patterns within the family. There are some concerns about its poor specificity to detect wake after sleep onset and applicability for children with movement disorders. It can be particularly useful in clinical practice in an '*n*-of-one' trial format when used to compare a period of time off medication with periods on different doses to optimize treatment
- PSG (with or without full EEG), while the gold standard for the diagnosis of many sleep disorders, is expensive, only available at a few specialist centres, and is neither practical nor accurate to use to track changes in sleep quantity or quality over time.

Magnitude of objective change

There is still lack of agreement about what sleep measure matters the most:

- At times, the best choice of parameter will be quite simple; if, e.g. the only problem is falling asleep, then sleep latency is the obvious outcome
- The most suitable parameter to capture the impact of night wakings is more difficult. There is a huge difference between ten wakings between 11 pm and midnight, and ten wakings that occur every hour of the night
- Sleep efficiency is sometimes used, but there is a lack of standardization on how it is recorded, and how much change matters
- A more recent measure, 'longest sleep period', shows promise as being responsive to change, and correlates with changes in the child's behaviours and the parent's quality of life.

Table 22.1 attempts to summarize common variables that are often used (based on sleep diaries or actigraphy), and what seems to be a clinically meaningful degree of change on which to plan treatment evaluations.

Table 22.1 Summary of common variables

Measure (units)	Clinical goal (significant degree of change)	Background rationale
Sleep onset latency (minutes)	Aim for minimum 15 minutes improvement and latency <30 minutes	Parent focus group work and consensus (Gringras et al., 2012)
Total sleep time (minutes)	Aim for minimum 45 minutes improvement	Work by Sadeh on sleep restriction and extension in children
Wake after sleep onset (minutes)	Huge variation: significant change 35 minutes	Normative PSG (Scholle et al., 2011)
Sleep efficiency (%)	Aim for >85% (significant change 6%)	Normative PSG (Scholle et al., 2011)
Longest sleep period	Aim for minimum 45 minutes improvement	Based on 0.5 standard deviation of the health-related quality of life (Gringras et al., 2017; Scholle et al., 2011)

General treatment approaches

Current guidance on management of insomnia-type sleep problems in children proposes that once physiological reasons for sleep disturbance are excluded, interventions that aim to change parents' management of their child's sleep should be the 'first port of call'. This guidance is also applicable to children with neurodisability, although the evidence for the effectiveness of behavioural interventions alone is less strong. Pharmacological interventions (such as melatonin) are recommended where such interventions prove ineffective or alongside parent-directed approaches.

Exclude physical and pharmacological sleep disruptors

It is important to consider the usual range of medical and pharmacological causes of sleep problems in this population before assuming there is a discrete insomnia related to the neurodisability. Because of difficulty identifying such 'sleep disruptors' in this often non-verbal population, there are some particular factors worthy of specific consideration.

Pain

Muscle spasm and joints

- Pain from muscle spasm or joints is common in young people with cerebral palsy and other movement disorders, and frequently underestimated or missed
- A range of pharmacological muscle relaxants are available and when unsuccessful, surgical interventions may be required
- Successful treatment of, e.g. adductor spasm with botulinum toxin injections is well documented as improving both pain scores and sleep quality.

Reflux and constipation

- Reflux and constipation are more common in virtually all children with neurodisability, and the pain and discomfort they cause is invariably worse at night
- Physical examination, X-rays, and abdominal ultrasound can help with accurate diagnosis
- Constipation needs to be properly treated and treatment continued for a long period of time to prevent recurrence
- Reflux is also more common in children with many neurodisabilities and pH impedance studies are probably the most helpful investigation of choice for possible acid or non-acid reflux in these children
- The reflux will be worse at night when lying down, and can cause pain, cough, or even central apnoea. The treatment of the reflux, whether pharmacological or surgical can often dramatically improve sleep.

ENT and dental

- While all ENT and dental problems can also occur in typically developing children, difficulties in communication with some non-verbal children with neurodisability can make examination and effective management more difficult
- At times, an empirical approach is taken, but examinations should not be withheld if required, even if hospital admission is required and investigations might require general anaesthesia.

Medication
- Children with neurodisability are often on complex combinations of centrally acting medications to reduce tone, seizures, or challenging behaviours
- There are no 'neutral' medications and all may have a direct or indirect impact on sleep
- Some specific examples will be discussed in ➲ Specific neurodisabilities, p. 238.

Comorbid physiological sleep disorders
- Many sleep disorders already described in typically developing children are seen more commonly in children with neurodisability due to a range of factors; e.g. OSA is more commonly associated with neurodisability for reasons including low muscle tone, craniofacial morphology, or obesity, or secondary to sedating medications
- Formal PSG is sometimes required for accurate diagnosis of sleep disorders and while such investigations might be challenging to perform, if anything a lower threshold is recommended for this population
- Ambulatory monitoring should be considered if inpatient sleep investigations are not possible.

Behavioural interventions
Parent-directed behavioural sleep interventions are always the first-line approach when treating insomnia in children with neurodisability.

Although there are some differences in approach based on the young person's level of understanding, and additional medical risks (such as nocturnal seizures), the general underlying principles remain the same as those already described in ➲ Chapter 20, although the evidence base is weaker.

In this group of families, who are often exhausted and at their wits' end, it is important to explain that such behavioural interventions can be as powerful as sleep medications, without the risk of adverse effects.

Pharmacological interventions
The use of most pharmacological interventions for paediatric sleep disorders lacks a robust evidence base and the majority of medications will be used unlicensed or off-label. Studies have been small and poorly controlled, although the situation is slowly improving. However, this provides little solace to a desperate family having to cope with a child's intolerable sleep problems, often without the resources to obtain respite or behavioural support.

The section that follows gives a brief overview of medications sometimes used in the management of insomnia-type sleep problems in children with neurodisability.

Melatonin
- A growing body of evidence indicates abnormal melatonin secretion and circadian rhythmicity in children with neurodevelopmental disorders, specifically autism spectrum disorder (ASD), which may explain the abnormal development of sleep–wake cycles, present from the first year of life
- Melatonin has the most extensive evidence base and a paediatric prolonged-release preparation is now licensed for children with ASD

- Robust studies supporting its use in children with ASD and ADHD and other neurodisabilities
- Typical doses: 0.5–10 mg
- Commoner adverse effects: changes in mood, drowsiness, and hangover effect.

Antihistamines

- Sedative side effects of antihistamines have long been used for childhood insomnia and sedation
- Over short periods, may improve sleep and speed up sleep behavioural programmes
- Some children can develop dramatic and paradoxical over-arousal
- Tolerance can develop quickly, and so they are usually effective only for short-term use
- Commoner adverse effects: dry mouth, drowsiness, and dizziness.

Chloral hydrate

- Previously popular hypnotic for children, but active metabolites have a very long half-life and considerable potential for 'hangover' effects in children
- It is now mainly used for sedation during diagnostic procedures
- Commoner adverse effects: paradoxical excitement, persistent drowsiness, and ataxia.

Clonidine

- Clonidine is an alpha-2 receptor agonist commonly used to treat hypertension, but also has sedative effects
- Typical doses: 25–125 micrograms
- In higher doses, clonidine leads to REM suppression and REM rebound with discontinuation
- Clonidine has been widely used in paediatric patients with ADHD and/or neurocognitive impairments and sleep disorders but with very limited published evidence
- Commoner adverse effects: hypotension, rebound hypertension, bradycardia or tachycardia, irritability, dysphoria, dizziness, headache, gastrointestinal effects, and dry mouth.

Benzodiazepines and non-benzodiazepine hypnotics

- Benzodiazepines and newer non-benzodiazepine 'Z drugs' such as zolpidem, zopiclone, and zaleplon, can shorten sleep latency and decrease awakenings for adults
- The most commonly used benzodiazepine for sleep in children is clonazepam, used mainly for arousal parasomnias such as sleep walking and sleep terrors in children
- There is no convincing paediatric data to support the use of benzodiazepines or 'Z drugs' for children and young people, who seem to be particularly sensitive to adverse effects including daytime behavioural disinhibition, ataxia, and amnesia.

Antidepressants

Tricyclic antidepressants are potent REM sleep suppressants and suppress SWS. Although previously used for children, concern about cardiac and other side effects, and other options, has reduced prescribing for this group.

Trazodone is a sedating 5-HT$_2$ receptor antagonist antidepressant often used second or third line for children with refractory insomnia:
- Typical doses 25–50 mg
- Commoner adverse effects of trazodone: dry mouth, blurred vision, dizziness, headache, and gastrointestinal effects. Although very rare, the risk of priapism is important and needs discussion where appropriate.

Specific neurodisabilities

Whether certain syndromes cause 'worse' or 'different' sleep difficulties is still uncertain. Identifying sleep 'endophenotypes' (profiles) for different syndromes may help understand aetiology, and tailor treatments. At present, such understanding is limited by low numbers, individual variation, sleep measurement inconsistency, and difficulty adjusting for underlying factors such as level of intellectual disability and seizures. Despite this, there do seem to be specific patterns that 'run true' and there is growing interest in comparisons cross-group.

Children with autism

Background
- Around 1% of children have an ASD
- Causes are still unclear and are likely to reflect a combination of a genetic predisposition, together with environmental or other unknown factors.

Sleep issues
- Children with an ASD are more likely to have disturbed sleep than typically developing children, with a prevalence of sleep disturbance in children with ASD around 70%
- The most common complaints are difficulties falling asleep and difficulties maintaining sleep. These difficulties persist from infancy throughout adult life
- The impact of such sleep problems is of particular concern given the increased burden and stress experienced in parenting a child with an ASD, and the potentially adverse effects of sleep disturbances and insufficient sleep on the child's and carers' daytime behaviour and cognitive functioning
- Comorbidity is the rule rather than the exception, and it is necessary to appreciate the often-additive contributions of common comorbidities such as ADHD, learning difficulties, tics, and seizures, all of which have their own independent effects on sleep
- This situation is further complicated as children with ASD and poor sleep demonstrate significantly higher daytime behavioural problems including irritability, and externalizing behaviours (specifically hyperactivity and aggression), compared to those who sleep well
- There is evidence to support a behavioural intervention both before a trial of melatonin (many will respond without requiring melatonin) and continuing a behavioural intervention while administering melatonin (the combination of both has been shown to be more effective than either one alone)
- The most recent randomized controlled study showed a paediatric mini-pill sustained-release melatonin was well tolerated, efficacious, and safe compared to placebo for treatment of insomnia in children with ASD
- This product, now licensed for treatment of insomnia in children with ASD, showed clinically meaningful improvements in total sleep time, duration of uninterrupted sleep (longest sleep episode), and sleep latency with corresponding behavioural improvements for the children, and improved quality of life measures in their parents over a 2-year period.

Children with attention deficit hyperactivity disorder

Background

- ADHD is described in 3–5% of children and young people, with boys more commonly affected
- Many of the behavioural and cognitive problems produced by poor quantity and quality of sleep in children overlap with those described in ADHD. Again, comorbidity is the rule, and ASD, learning difficulties, tics, and seizures can coexist
- ADHD is best understood as a '24/7' disorder, where the same impulsivity and motor restlessness seen during the day is likely to manifest during the night as well.

Sleep issues

- As the sleep difficulties may often precede formal ADHD diagnosis, there is a 'chicken and egg' debate about the relationship between the two
- In 75% of ADHD patients, the physiological sleep phase, where people show the physiological signs associated with sleep, such as changes in the level of the sleep hormone melatonin, core body temperature, and changes in sleep-related movement are all delayed
- A number of sleep disorders are associated with ADHD, including RLS, sleep apnoea, and delayed sleep phase syndrome
- In keeping with treatment of ASD, melatonin, behavioural interventions, and parent education/interventions appear to be the most effective strategies to improve multiple domains of sleep problems
- Two randomized controlled trials showed the effectiveness of melatonin for children with ADHD, most specifically in reducing sleep latency
- In children with ADHD, the daytime management of the ADHD is often important and often an '*n*-of-one' trial of altering medications over time for an individual child is required
- Broadly speaking, stimulant medications which form the bedrock of ADHD treatment can increase sleep latency significantly for some children. However, there are a number of situations where a small dose of an immediate-release stimulant given in the evening will paradoxically allow a young person's level of hyper-aroused behaviours to calm down and facilitate easier bedtime settling
- Some medications used for daytime management of ADHD symptoms are less likely to lengthen sleep latency (e.g. atomoxetine), while others can even increase sleepiness and improve sleep latency and at times sleep efficiency (e.g. clonidine and guanfacine)
- Thus, the management of sleep issues in young people with ADHD is complex, and often requires careful consideration of multiple medications and their individual effects on sleep.

Children with epilepsy

Background

Epilepsy-specific quality of life in children and young people is not determined solely by seizures, but rather by factors such as a child's learning, mental health, sleep, and social support.

Sleep issues
- There are a number of seizure disorders almost exclusively associated with sleep
- Nocturnal seizures can interrupt sleep while a number of factors, including antiepileptics and sleep disorders, that cause sleep fragmentation can worsen seizures
- Antiepileptic drugs, as well as other non-pharmacological epilepsy interventions, can all affect sleep quality
- Parent-led behavioural sleep interventions are underused and have potential to improve sleep of children, and their families.

See also ➲ Chapter 25.

Children with cerebral palsy

Background
Cerebral palsy is the name for a group of lifelong conditions that affect movement, posture, and coordination, usually caused by an injury to the brain that occurs before, during, or soon after birth.

Sleep issues
- The associated intellectual, seizure, and motor difficulties in this group of children mean that 'typical sleep patterns' are rarely experienced by caregivers for this particular group
- Consider physical causes or pain and discomfort (reflux, muscle spasm, hip pain)
- Sleep apnoea should be excluded
- Pharmacological approaches are complicated by multiple day and night-time medications
- There is a tendency for high doses of sedating medications to be used; unfortunately, tolerance can develop rapidly, and it can be difficult to differentiate adverse effects of medications from difficulties related to the condition itself.

Children with Down syndrome

Background
- Down syndrome is the most common genetic cause of intellectual disability, with an incidence of 1 in 691 live births caused when an error in cell division results in an extra chromosome 21
- There can be impairments in cognitive ability and physical growth, mild to moderate developmental disabilities, and a higher risk of some health problems.

Sleep issues
- Children with Down syndrome have craniofacial features, including mid-facial hypoplasia, narrow nasopharynx, micrognathia, small larynx, large tongue, and hypotonia leading to floppiness of the upper airways, that increase their risk of having SDB issues, particularly OSA
- As ~50% have OSA, and there are no reliable diagnostic questionnaires, formal inpatient or ambulatory testing for OSA is recommended in all cases
- Children also experience more night-time awakenings, lower overall sleep time, and lower quality sleep overall, with more time in stage 1 sleep and less time in more restorative sleep

- Children with Down syndrome also have greater resistance to and anxiety around bedtime than their peers without Down syndrome, with 66% falling asleep in a parent's or sibling's bed. Almost 20% wake up early, and 40% wake at least once during the night
- Behavioural strategies, sometimes in combination with melatonin to reduce sleep latency, can be helpful.

Smith–Magenis syndrome

Background

- Smith–Magenis syndrome is characterized by multiple congenital anomalies and a well-defined, severe pattern behaviour problems, including self-injury and abnormal sleep patterns
- Most commonly due to a 3.5 Mb interstitial deletion of chromosome 17 band p11.2.

Sleep issues

- Published reports of 24-hour melatonin secretion patterns document an inverted endogenous melatonin pattern in virtually all cases
- Children with Smith–Magenis syndrome display difficulties getting to sleep, frequent nocturnal awakenings, early sleep offset, and daytime sleepiness with a need for daytime naps
- There is increased risk of associated airway abnormalities and so the potential for OSA needs consideration and investigation if required
- Trials suggest that when an inverted melatonin rhythm exists there is benefit from combined use of morning beta-blockers (acebutolol 10 mg/kg) and evening melatonin
- This combination can inhibit daytime melatonin production and maintain daytime alertness, improving sleep consolidation at night, and may result in some behavioural improvements.

Angelman syndrome

Background

- Angelman syndrome is a neurogenetic condition characterized by developmental delay, absence of speech, motor impairment, epilepsy, and a characteristic behavioural phenotype that includes sleep problems
- It is caused by lack of expression of the *UBE3A* gene on the maternal chromosome 15q11–q13.

Sleep issues

- Reduced total sleep time, increased sleep onset latency, disrupted sleep architecture with frequent nocturnal awakenings, reduced REM sleep, and periodic leg movements
- Interaction between sleep and seizures can be important
- Management may be difficult, particularly in young children; it primarily involves behavioural approaches, though pharmacological treatment may be required. Medications require specialist supervision as the risk of poor sleep needs balancing against the risk of worsening seizure control:
  - Anecdotally melatonin is rarely effective—decreased sleep duration and increased sleep fragmentation are the most dominant features
  - Clonidine is also rarely effective, whereas trazodone seems particularly effective.

Rett syndrome

Background

- Rett syndrome is a severe neurological disorder, affecting mainly females. It is generally caused by mutations in the *MECP2* gene
- The prevalence of sleep problems seems to be highest in cases with a large deletion of the *MECP2* gene and in those with the p.R294X or p.R306C mutations.

Sleep issues

- Sleep problems occur in >80% of cases
- Night waking is dominated by night-time laughter and night screaming
- The prevalence of night-time laughter and night screaming decreases with age, while reported night-time seizures and daytime napping increases with age
- There are no evidence-based specific treatments although complex autonomic testing is proposed to better understand different breathing and arousal phenotypes
- EEG video-telemetry is often required to identify the relative contributions of seizures or sleep-related breathing triggers.

Williams syndrome

Background

- Williams syndrome is a developmental disorder caused by a microdeletion in a distinct region of chromosome 7 (7q11.23)
- Prevalence is estimated at 1 in 7500
- Patients manifest a variety of major phenotypic features, including neurological, neurocognitive, cardiovascular, musculoskeletal, and endocrine abnormalities.

Sleep issues

- Sleep efficiency is significantly decreased in patients compared to controls
- Although a small study showed an association between Williams syndrome and periodic limb movements, this was not borne out by a subsequent larger study
- Williams syndrome subjects have more frequent respiratory-related arousals than controls
- Overnight PSG can be useful in excluding comorbid physiological sleep disorders.

Tuberous sclerosis

Background

- Tuberous sclerosis complex (TSC) is a genetic disorder affecting 1 in 6000 live births, and is caused by mutations in the tumour suppressor genes *TSC1* or *TSC2*
- In TSC, mutations in these genes lead to benign tumours affecting multiple organs, including the skin, kidneys, and heart
- In >90% of patients, the brain is involved often resulting in significant morbidity including seizures, intellectual disability, autism, ADHD, depression, and anxiety
- Seizure disorders occur in 70–90% of patients with TSC, most often presenting in the first year of life.

Sleep issues

- In children with TSC, severe sleep problems can often be due to sleep-related epileptic events
- PSG studies show that children with TSC and seizures have a more disturbed sleep architecture than those who do not have seizures
- Sleep disorders, including night waking, early waking, seizure-related sleep problems, and EDS, have previously been recognized as a frequent cause and result of stress in the more severely affected patients with TSC and their families
- Melatonin can be helpful if sleep onset is prolonged.

Further reading

For patients

Autism Speaks Sleep Toolkit. Available at: 🔗 https://www.autismspeaks.org/science/resources-programs/autism-treatment-network/tools-you-can-use/sleep-tool-kit

Raising Children Network: ADHD and Sleep. Available at: 🔗 http://raisingchildren.net.au/articles/adhd.html

For clinicians

Boban S, Leonard H, Wong K, et al. Sleep disturbances in Rett syndrome: impact and management including use of sleep hygiene practices. Am J Med Genet A. 2018;176(7):1569–77.

Cortesi F, Giannotti F, Sebastiani T, et al. Controlled-release melatonin, singly and combined with cognitive behavioural therapy, for persistent insomnia in children with autism spectrum disorders: a randomized placebo-controlled trial. J Sleep Res. 2012;21(6):700–709.

Gibbon F, Maccormac E, Gringras P. Sleep and epilepsy: unfortunate bedfellows. Arch Dis Child. 2019; 104(2):189–92.

Gringras P. When to use drugs to help sleep. Arch Dis Child. 2008;93:976–81.

Gringras P, Gamble C, Jones A. Melatonin for sleep problems in children with neurodevelopmental disorders: randomised double masked placebo controlled trial. BMJ. 2012;345:e6664.

Gringras P, Nir T, Breddy J, et al. Efficacy and safety of pediatric prolonged-release melatonin for insomnia in children with autism spectrum disorder. J Am Acad Child Adolesc Psychiatry. 2017;56(11):948–57.

Mindell JA, Owen J. A Clinical Guide to Pediatric Sleep: Diagnosis and Management of Sleep Problems, 3rd ed. Philadelphia, PA: Lippincott Williams & Wilkins; 2015.

Raising Children Network. ADHD and Sleep. Available at: 🔗 http://raisingchildren.net.au/articles/adhd.html

Sadeh A. The role and validity of actigraphy in sleep medicine: an update. Sleep Medicine Reviews. 2011;15(4):259–67.

Scholle S, Beyer U, Bernhard M, et al. Normative values of polysomnographic parameters in childhood and adolescence: quantitative sleep parameters. Sleep Med. 2011;12(6):542–9.

Taylor D, Paton C, Kapur S (Eds). Maudsley Prescribing Guidelines, 10th ed. London: Informa Healthcare; 2009. Available at: 🔗 http://fac.ksu.edu.sa/sites/default/files/Prescribing_Guidelines11.pdf

Van der Heijden KB, Smits MG, Van Someren EJ, et al. Effect of melatonin on sleep, behavior, and cognition in ADHD and chronic sleep-onset insomnia. J Am Acad Child Adolesc Psychiatry. 2007;46(2):233–41.

Sleep and cognition

Ivana Rosenzweig, Michelle Olaithe,
Romola S. Bucks, and Mary J. Morrell

Introduction

Sleep is a brain phenomenon, and the principal role for sleep in a number of cognitive and emotional processes is increasingly well understood. Such cognitive processes include neural oscillations and synchronization among brain regions that are active during attention, perception, working memory, short- and long-term memory acquisition, retention and recall, imagination, and thought.

Over the last few decades, clinicians, epidemiologists, and neuroscientists have documented significant associations between the severity of sleep disturbance and the degree of impairment of selective cognitive functions, in a variety of clinical populations. Of particular clinical note is that sleep disorder and associated cognitive deficits may be one of the earliest signs of neurodegenerative disorders, including early AD and PD.

Sleep is likely to play an important role in numerous functions related to cognitive abilities, including:

- *Memory processing and brain plasticity*—sleep has been implicated in the encoding and consolidation of memory, both of which are required for memories to persist over the longer time course
- *The glymphatic system* refers to a recently discovered macroscopic waste clearance system that utilizes a unique system of perivascular channels, formed by astroglial cells, to promote efficient elimination of soluble proteins and metabolites from the central nervous system. Apart from waste elimination, the glymphatic system may also function to help distribute non-waste compounds, such as glucose, lipids, amino acids, and neurotransmitters. The glymphatic system functions mainly during sleep and is largely disengaged during wakefulness. It has been suggested that during SWS, elimination of potentially neurotoxic waste products, including beta-amyloid, occurs via the glymphatic system.

Presently, two models of sleep-dependent plasticity relevant to declarative memory are used to explain the overnight facilitation of recall:

1. Hippocampal–neocortical dialogue, where sleep, in particular SWS, facilitates the shift of information from short-term storage to long-term storage within neocortical circuits
2. Synaptic homeostasis hypothesis, where SWS promotes a decrease in synaptic connections occurring in wakefulness, thus maintaining plasticity, and REM sleep provides a neural environment in which the synaptic remodelling of neural circuitry essential to learning and cognition occurs.

Clinical features

Sleep quality, quantity, and cognition

Either shorter or longer durations of sleep than those advised for the particular neurodevelopmental stage can be associated with poorer cognitive function:

- Adverse changes in sleep duration over time are shown to be linked to lower scores on a variety of cognitive function tests, excluding memory function
- People who sleep for 11 hours or more per night have significantly lower global cognition scores than those who sleep for 7 hours
- A short nap has been found to improve alertness, sleepiness, short-term memory, and accuracy, but it has not been shown to affect reaction times
- Very little research has been done to explore the effects of subtle changes in circadian phase on cognition (e.g. weekend binge sleep, daylight saving time). However, one study has revealed that performance on memory and verbal fluency tasks is significantly reduced following delayed weekend sleep
- It is broadly accepted that proper alignment between homeostatic and circadian time is crucial for cognitive performance
- The deficits in daytime performance due to sleep loss are associated with a significant socioeconomic, societal, and individual human cost
- There are two major types of sleep loss: acute sleep loss (e.g. one continuous extended wake episode) and chronic sleep loss (e.g. consisting of insufficient sleep over multiple days).

Practical clinical considerations

The cognitive impact of short-term total sleep deprivation (<48 hours) includes the following:

- Tasks of greater complexity are initially less susceptible to the effects of total sleep deprivation
- Simple attention or vigilance are shown to be most strongly affected
- Significant implications for occupational and driving fitness have been suggested, where deficits in sustained and divided attention likely act as an early warning for subsequent cognitive failure in more complex skills
- Sleep debt can be expressed as additional wakefulness that has the cost of cognitive impairment, and which accumulates over time
- Sleep homeostatic physiological processes can replenish this capacity, but it is not clear how much sleep is required to ameliorate previous sleep debt
- Neuroimaging evidence has implicated the frontal and parietal cortex as brain regions that may be particularly susceptible to the effects of sleep loss
- Emerging evidence suggests that some aspects of higher-level cognitive capacities remain degraded by sleep deprivation despite restoration of alertness and vigilance with stimulant countermeasures, suggesting that sleep loss may affect specific cognitive systems above and beyond the effects produced by global cognitive declines or impaired attentional processes
- Sleep deprivation may also particularly affect cognitive systems that rely on emotional data.

Thus, the extent to which sleep deprivation affects a particular cognitive process likely depends on several factors, including the global decline in attention, the degree to which the specific cognitive function depends on emotion-processing networks, and the extent to which that cognitive process can draw upon associated regions for compensatory support.

Sleep quality, or how well we actually sleep during the night, also plays an important role in cognition and disturbed sleep is strongly associated with an increased risk of developing a cognitive impairment.

Sleep in older age

Normal ageing is associated with reduced ability to initiate and maintain sleep. Physiological adult age-dependent changes in sleep, unlike those of childhood, are relatively well known, and include changes in sleep architecture, increased sleep fragmentation, and increased susceptibility to certain sleep disorders, such as OSA, insomnia, and RBD. Advancing beyond the fifth decade of age is associated with several well-characterized changes in sleep architecture:

- Advanced sleep timing (i.e. earlier bedtimes and rise times)
- Longer sleep onset latency (i.e. longer time taken to fall asleep)
- Shorter overall sleep duration
- Increased sleep fragmentation (i.e. less consolidated sleep with more awakenings, arousals, or transitions to lighter sleep stages)
- More fragile sleep (i.e. higher likelihood of being woken by external sensory stimuli)
- Reduced amount of SWS
- Increased time spent in lighter NREM stages 1 and 2
- Shorter and fewer NREM–REM sleep cycles
- Increased time spent awake throughout the night
- Sex and gender differences in sleep changes have been well documented. The majority of sleep changes are more prominent in men, but this changes in women post menopause (see following section)
- The frequency of diurnal naps also increases in later life: 10% of adults aged 55–64 years, and 25% of those aged 75–84 years, report the occurrence of daytime naps. The Medical Research Council Cognitive Function and Ageing Study (CFAS) found that daytime napping at baseline is associated with a lower risk of cognitive decline at 2- and 10-year follow-ups. In addition, reports of both EDS and obtaining <6.5 hours of night-time sleep are associated with an increased risk of cognitive decline at 10-year follow-up.

Peri- and postmenopausal changes

Sleep is modulated by ovarian hormones in women across the adult lifespan. Loss of ovarian function in women is associated with sleep disturbances and cognitive decline, which suggest a key role for oestrogens and progestogens in modulating these symptoms. The effects of ovarian hormones on sleep and cognitive processes have been studied in separate research fields that seldom intersect. A growing body of evidence indicates that the development of sleep disorders following menopause contributes to accelerated cognitive decline and dementia in older women:

- The known effects of oestrogen-related central nervous system actions include increasing levels of neurotransmitters, enhancing neuron growth, and formation of synapses, acting as antioxidant and regulatory effects on calcium homeostasis and second messenger systems
- Sleep complaints increase during periods of large fluctuations of ovarian hormones, including puberty, pregnancy, and the menopausal transition
- There is also evidence for sleep changes across the menstrual cycle: poorest quality is reported during the mid-to-late luteal phase; this phase is associated with increased reports of night-time awakenings and arousals, and with decreased SWS

- Differences in objective sleep measures are also observed in women taking oral contraceptives as indicated by increased N2, REM, and reduced SWS relative to naturally cycling women.

About 40–60% of perimenopausal women report sleep disturbances and insomnia. The menopausal transition is associated with increased frequency of self-reported problems, such as falling and staying asleep and reduced total sleep time:

- A critical determinant of the effects of oestrogen on the CNS, including on sleep and cognition, appears to be the timing of oestrogen exposure in relation to the menopausal transition and age. In the case of cognitive outcomes, some evidence supports the 'critical window hypothesis' implying that exposure early in the menopausal transition or postmenopausal period confers cognitive benefit, whereas exposure later in the menopausal transition may have no or even detrimental effects
- Levels of follicle-stimulating hormone may also play a role in sleep quality, as they are positively related to waking after sleep onset, number of awakenings, and arousals in perimenopausal women without sleep complaints
- Disturbed sleep architecture during perimenopausal changes has been linked to the presence of vasomotor symptoms (hot flushes) and lower sleep efficiency and more sleep complaints
- Higher cortisol levels or greater cortisol reactivity may be one mechanism that links hot flushes, sleep, and depression or anxiety symptoms to decrements in cognitive performance. Cortisol increases after a hot flush, experimental administration of corticosteroids produces verbal memory impairment, and higher endogenous cortisol levels are associated with poorer performance on memory tasks. It has been suggested that oestrogen replacement therapy may buffer this stress response
- OSA prevalence increases markedly at menopause, partly due to weight gain, and, although unclear, also to hormone changes and other mechanisms
- Menopausal sleep disruption can exacerbate other pre-existing sleep disorders, including RLS and circadian disorders
- Also, higher risks of insomnia and depressive and anxiety disorders have been reported
- Postmenopausal women with hormone replacement therapy have a reduced latency to fall asleep and fewer night-time awakenings and wakefulness
- Oestradiol given for 8 weeks to peri- and postmenopausal women is associated with reduced self-reported insomnia symptoms and improved sleep quality
- Antidepressant and hormonal replacement therapy may play a significant therapeutic role, especially in the early stages of hormonal changes. However, the exact mechanisms are unclear.

Sleep disorders and cognition

Findings from observational studies support a role for sleep disturbances (e.g. duration, fragmentation, and OSA) in the development of cognitive impairment. The evidence is less clear for the association of insomnia and circadian rhythm dysfunction with cognition:

• Patients with OSA have been shown to suffer with deficits in cognitive domains of attention and vigilance, long-term (episodic), verbal and visual memory, and visuospatial or constructional abilities
• All aspects of executive functioning can be affected in OSA patients, including the ability to shift between tasks or mental sets, to inhibit dominant responses, in updating and monitoring working memory representations, in efficiently accessing semantic stores, fluid reasoning, or problem-solving
• Information processing and fine motor control may be reduced
• There is less consistent evidence of short-term memory deficits, or of notable problems with expressive or receptive language
• Conversion to mild cognitive impairment (MCI) and AD may occur at a younger age
• Treating OSA with CPAP may delay the age of onset of MCI and improve cognitive function in AD
• Patients with AD may have a five times higher risk of OSA
• About 50% of patients with AD will have experienced OSA at some time after their initial diagnosis, negatively impacting its prognosis and quality of life.

Sleep and dementia

Alzheimer's disease

Other neurodegenerative disorders

Parkinson's disease

Sleep and dementia

Sleep disruption constitutes a core component of most neurodegenerative processes, and signature abnormalities of sleep have been shown to emerge well before clinical onset of many dementias.

Although increased prevalence of sleep disturbances in people with dementia has been well documented, and it is often thought to result from neurodegeneration, focus has turned towards the possibility that sleep disturbances can also increase the risk of cognitive decline and dementia. The sleep–wake cycle is regulated by complex interactions among brain regions and neurotransmitter systems, which are implicated in memory and cognitive function. In view of this shared circuitry, sleep problems are not just common in people with AD and other dementias, but likely contribute to, and shape the disease process.

Alzheimer's disease

Significant correlations between subjective and objective measures of poor sleep with the severity of cortical amyloid-beta burden, CSF measures of amyloid-beta, and phosphorylated tau in CSF have been demonstrated in cognitively normal older adults, MCI, and AD patients.

Similarly, the hypocretin/orexinergic system is shown to be dysregulated in AD, where its output and function appears to be overexpressed along the progression of the neurodegenerative process.

The prevalence of sleep disturbance in AD has been estimated to be 25% in mild to moderate cases, and up to 50% in moderate to severe cases.

In adults with AD, circadian rhythm dysfunction and so-called sundowning (increased confusion and restlessness at the end of the day and into the night) are frequently reported, and they are thought to result from degeneration of the suprachiasmatic nucleus and the cholinergic neurons of the nucleus basalis of Meynert.

In the community setting, patients with mild to moderate AD are frequently reported to suffer from insomnia and fragmented sleep during the night and excessive sleeping during daytime, the intensity of which correlates with the severity of dementia.

Patients with amnestic MCI show EEG abnormalities, including fewer sleep spindles and reduced SWS.

Similar sleep impairments are also present in older adults who are carriers of the ε4 allele of the apolipoprotein E (*APOE*) gene. A higher *APOE-ε*4 dose is associated with greater cognitive impairment.

Reduced amount, delayed onset, and blunted rebound of REM sleep following selective deprivation can occur in patients with MCI and AD.

Reductions in the EEG quality of REM sleep have been proposed as a possible biomarker that could help discriminate those with AD from cognitively normal older adults.

Other neurodegenerative disorders

Parkinson's disease

- Approximately 80% of non-demented PD patients develop dementia within 8 years
- REM sleep reduction may trigger hallucinations by enabling the emergence of REM sleep during wakefulness

- Hallucinations have been significantly correlated with the presence of RBD, independently of age, sex, and disease duration, but related to the amount of dopaminergic medication
- RBD is an early manifestation of a neurodegenerative synucleinopathy (e.g. DLB, PD, and multiple system atrophy)—see ➲ Chapter 18
- One-third of patients with PD present with EEG slowing regardless of the presence of dementia.

Dementia with Lewy bodies
- Significant sleep disturbances, daytime somnolence, and sleep-related movement disorders
- Normal hypocretin/orexin levels
- OSA might occur in up to 88% and PLMS in up to 74% of patients
- Poor sleep efficiency.

Vascular dementia
- Patients with vascular dementia have a significantly greater disruption of sleep–wake cycles associated with poor sleep quality than those with AD
- No correlation between the degree of sleep disruption and the severity of intellectual deterioration has been identified
- There is a strong association with OSA
- Larger EEG source fluctuations than in AD have been reported, reflecting decreased vigilance and increased fluctuations in cognition.

Frontotemporal dementia
- Accompanied by a disturbance of the homeostatic and of the sleep–wake rhythm
- EEG slowing during wakefulness.

Progressive supranuclear palsy
- EDS is common
- Orexin levels can be low, and inversely correlated with the duration of the illness
- Absence or drastic reduction of REM sleep is commonly observed with progression of the illness; there is a correlation with a decline in cognitive functioning
- Positive association between degree of impairment on frontal cognitive tasks and EEG slowing.

Creutzfeldt–Jakob disease
- A hallmark of wake EEG is the presence of periodic sharp wave complexes within a background of generalized slow and low-voltage EEG, suggestive of diffuse pathology (present in two-thirds of patients with CJD, and only in 9% of other disorders)
- Disorganized sleep patterns, sudden jumps between stages
- Very few sleep spindles and K-complexes (N2)
- Absence or significant decrease of N3 stage
- A lower REM percentage and REM density.

Potential therapeutic options

Therapeutic interventions that can modulate NREM SWS (e.g. auditory closed-loop stimulation or transcranial current stimulation) might, in future, be used as a preventative measure to reduce AD risk in younger patients, or in high-vulnerability populations, such as patients with Down syndrome or individuals carrying the *APOE-ε4* allele with marked sleep deficits. Similarly, cholinesterase inhibitors have been shown to increase REM sleep quality and duration and they also help with memory, mood, and emotional symptoms in some dementia patients.

Currently, however, the staple treatment of sleep disturbances in patients with dementia does not differ from that in other age groups, and it consists of predominantly focusing on treating any underlying sleep disorder, such as described in other chapters.

Further reading

Bernier A, Beauchamp MH, Bouvette-Turcot AA, et al. Sleep and cognition in preschool years: specific links to executive functioning. Child Dev. 2013; 84 (5):1542–53.

Bucks RS, Olaithe M, Rosenzweig I, et al. Reviewing the relationship between OSA and cognition: where do we go from here? Respirology. 2017;22(7):1253–61.

Killgore WD. Effects of sleep deprivation on cognition. Prog Brain Res. 2010;185:105–29.

Krause AJ, Simon EB, Mander BA, et al. The sleep-deprived human brain. Nat Rev Neurosci. 2017;18(7):404–18.

Sleep and headache disorders

Alexander D. Nesbitt

Introduction

Sleep problems and headache are among the most common symptoms we experience. It is no surprise that some co-associations between the two exist, although quite how the interactions occur are complex, and quite elusive. There are many layers of considerable overlap in terms of the anatomy, physiology, and pharmacology of the brain systems involved in headache and sleep–wake, but it is beyond the scope of this chapter to examine these.

Migraine

Migraine is the most common neurological disorder. Headache, which is the most recognized symptom of the syndrome, is typically throbbing, and accompanied by other symptoms including nausea (and vomiting) and sensory phobias (worsening of head pain with light, sound, smell, and movement). Some episodes include an aura phase before the headache, in which a spreading wave of neuronal depolarization fans out across the cerebral cortex, causing a series of symptoms, including visual, sensory, speech, and occasional motor and brainstem disturbances. Attacks typically last <72 hours.

A multifaceted association with sleep has long been noted, but the association is complex, and remains poorly understood. The levels of this relationship include:

- Sleep disturbance (too little > too much) being a strong trigger of migraine (second commonest after stress)
- Sleep disturbances may be an early (premonitory) feature of a migraine attack
- Overwhelming sleepiness rarely occurring as an aura symptom in migraine with brainstem aura
- Insomnia or sleepiness occasionally occurring as part of the 'postdrome' of an attack
- Sleep, particularly in children, having a therapeutic role in terminating an attack
- A history of childhood arousal parasomnias is a potential marker for having migraine.

The attacks of migraine are more likely to occur in the morning, which may be either a circadian or sleep homeostatic effect. Earlier chronotypes are slightly more likely to have migraine than later chronotypes, and this is borne out by the observation that patients with familial advanced sleep phase syndrome 2 (FASPS2) also have migraine with aura.

Longitudinal population studies derive consistent odds ratios of 1.7 for developing migraine in people with insomnia, and vice versa, over an 11-year period; rising to 2.2 odds ratio for developing insomnia with medium- to high-frequency migraine over the same period.

RLS also co-associates with migraine, with pooled cohort studies suggesting an odds ratio of 1.2.

Concomitant sleep disorders (chronic insomnia, OSA, PLMD, CRSWDs, NREM arousal parasomnias, idiopathic hypersomnia) are risk factors for developing chronic migraine, and should be assessed for and treated early, as treatment once chronic migraine has set in does not necessarily improve migraine.

Treatment of migraine can have a bearing on sleep. These relationships include:

- Reduction of melatonin amplitude with NSAID use
- Somnolence is a commonly reported adverse effect of triptan use, more so with central nervous system-penetrant triptans (eletriptan, zolmitriptan) and less so with less penetrant triptans (almotriptan, naratriptan)

- Propranolol, an often-used preventive medication, also reduces melatonin levels, and reduces the arousal threshold in REM sleep (giving rise to vivid dreams)
- Amitriptyline, another commonly used preventive, promotes drowsiness and therefore sleep, but is associated with often considerable sleep inertia, and can worsen RLS
- Melatonin is occasionally used as adjunct treatment in migraine, but often with only transient and limited success.

Standard advice for improving sleep behaviours is very important for patients with migraine, and CBT-I (with sleep compression therapy, rather than restriction therapy, which can worsen and trigger migraine) shows some anecdotal promise, both in terms of treating insomnia and also reducing frequency of episodic migraine.

Cluster headache

Attacks of cluster headache (CH) wake the majority of sufferers up from sleep nightly, usually at the same time, typically 60–90 minutes after sleep onset. Several attacks may occur during each major sleep episode. The majority of sufferers will also experience attacks during wake.

- Prevalence is 0.12%
- Men are more affected than women (2.5–3.5:1)
- Usual age of onset is in third to fifth decade
- About 70% of sufferers will be current or ex-smokers, but no clear causation exists
- The attacks are strictly unilateral, typically centred around the orbit and temple
- The pain is extreme ('11/10', 'worst pain ever', spearing, stabbing, burning)
- Ipsilateral to the pain, there is usually a varying combination of:
  - Ptosis
  - Conjunctival injection (redness)
  - Lacrimation
  - Nasal congestion and rhinorrhoea
  - Forehead sweating
  - Face swelling
  - Fullness of the ear
- In marked contrast to migraine, 90% of patients will be restless and agitated, and want to move about, pace, rock, or bang their heads.

The attacks start quickly, build in intensity rapidly, and last between 15 and 180 minutes. They occur between once every 48 hours, to eight times in 24 hours; classically at similar times each day. The majority of sufferers (50–75%) have both nocturnal sleep attacks and daytime attacks, but a proportion (20%) will only have nocturnal attacks. Attacks can also arise from longer daytime naps. Triggers include alcohol (small amounts inducing attacks within an hour of ingestion) and solvents (paint, perfumes).

Attacks 'cluster' together into bouts, lasting a mean of 8 weeks, and occurring on average once or twice a year, often at the same time of year, when photoperiod length is at its maximal rates of change, i.e. spring and autumn. Around 10% of sufferers have chronic CH, and have continuous attacks without any remission periods.

Functional imaging studies point to a role of posterior hypothalamic areas in CH attack pathogenesis, and various lines of enquiry have suggested some role of the hypocretin/orexin-ergic system, at least in modulating the attacks, but without any clear evidence. The sleep-arising attacks can occur from REM and NREM sleep, and do not appear to be associated with any clear sleep-related trigger.

Some studies have reported a higher incidence of OSA in patients with CH compared to the general population. However, treatment of OSA with PAP does not seem to prevent the attacks from occurring. Patients with chronic CH and OSA often find standard PAP facemasks uncomfortable to wear, and may prefer nasal pillow-style interfaces.

Various other sleep disorders and complaints can coexist, most notably chronic sleep loss from nocturnal attacks, resulting in daytime sleepiness, and in some cases insomnia (through fear of going to sleep). The incidence of comorbid RLS is unknown. These should be addressed where possible, to try and help mitigate the impact of sleep loss resulting from the attacks occurring at night.

High doses of melatonin (up to 15 mg) at night may be a useful adjunct helpful in treating the disorder (and, also at lower doses, the insomnia it can be associated with), but the evidence for this is thin. A small case series of patients with refractory chronic CH suggested nocturnal administration of sodium oxybate may be helpful, but this has not been systematically trialled.

Patients with CH should be under the care of a neurologist with an interest in headache disorders.

Treatment is aimed at aborting the individual attacks:
• Parenteral triptans, such as subcutaneous sumatriptan
• High-flow oxygen (12–15 L a minute for 15 minutes via a non-rebreather bag-mask)
• Providing temporary respite with greater occipital nerve blocks.

Prophylactic solutions include:
• Medication, such as verapamil, lithium, or topiramate
• Devices in patients with chronic CH (non-invasive vagus nerve stimulation; minimally invasive sphenopalatine ganglion stimulation).

Rarer, related disorders exist, which are also associated with attacks or exacerbations waking patients from sleep, and resulting in sleep loss and fragmentation. These include paroxysmal hemicrania, in which the attacks are essentially very similar, but shorter (2–30 minutes), and tend to occur more frequently (>5 in 24 hours). Hemicrania continua is continuous milder unilateral head pain resembling migraine, with extreme exacerbations resembling CH on top. Both can wake sufferers from sleep, but usually less regularly than CH might. Both paroxysmal hemicrania and hemicrania continua are very sensitive to prophylactic use of indomethacin daily. Indomethacin use can precipitate OSA, so regular enquiry and screening should be considered.

Hypnic headache

Hypnic headache is a very rare primary headache disorder, with attacks exclusively arising during, and waking patients from, sleep (typically nocturnal, but also daytime naps):

* Prevalence is unknown
* More common in people over the age of 50 years
* Patients are routinely woken (on >10 nights a month), typically 2–5 hours after sleep onset (i.e. later into the sleep episode than CH) by a mild to moderate (20% severe) dull, featureless headache (both sides or one sided), lasting 15–240 minutes
* Mild migrainous features (such as mild nausea) may be present in some patients, but is not typical.

Some studies have noted raised average AHIs (10 events/hour), but the presence of other primary sleep disorders does not necessarily rule out the diagnosis: it just complicates it.

MRI-based imaging studies have suggested volume loss in the posterior hypothalamic area in hypnic headache. Like CH, the attacks can occur in NREM and REM sleep, without any obvious triggers.

Assessment is by careful history taking and examination, with differentiation from, and exclusion of, other causes of nocturnal headache (➔ Secondary headaches, p. 266). Most would advocate MRI scanning, although the yield is likely to be low. PSG is helpful only for screening for comorbid sleep disorders, if suspected.

Treatment of hypnic headache is based largely on anecdotal reports, including using:

* Caffeine—both preventively before bed, and acutely (can precipitate insomnia)
* Indomethacin preventively before bed (can worsen OSA)
* Lithium (can worsen RLS)
* Melatonin (3–6 mg)
* Lamotrigine (few cases only).

Sleep apnoea headache

Morning headache is a well-recognized symptom of OSA. The International Classification of Headache Disorders (third edition) recognizes a clear, and distinct, headache phenotype associated with OSA. For this to be present:

- Sleep apnoea must have been diagnosed
- Evidence of causation must be demonstrated by at least two of the following:
  - Headache has developed in close temporal onset of OSA
  - Either or both of the following:
    - Headache has worsened in parallel with worsening of OSA
    - Headache has significantly improved/remitted in parallel with improvement/resolution of OSA
- Headache has at least one of the following three characteristics:
  - Recurs on >15 days a month
  - All of the following:
    - Bilateral
    - Pressing quality
    - Not accompanied by nausea, photophobia, or phonophobia
  - Resolves within 4 hours
- Not accounted for by another International Classification of Headache Disorders (third edition) diagnosis.

The prevalence of sleep apnoea headache among patients with OSA is 12–18%. Of interest, there is *no difference* in OSA parameters (AHI, saturation levels) between patients with and without sleep apnoea headache, meaning the long-held thought that headache must be related to oxygen and/or carbon dioxide levels is unlikely to be the pathophysiological mechanism driving the headache.

Exploding head syndrome

This phenomenon is covered in ➲ Chapter 19. It is mentioned here as there is a common misconception, given its dramatic name, that it represents a pain state, rather than a sensory misperception or sensory sleep start variant.

Bruxism

Bruxism is covered in ➲ Chapter 19. Bruxism can contribute to temporomandibular joint dysfunction, and pain in the jaw can radiate to the head. It can be treated with occlusal splints and MADs, although attempts are often unsatisfactory in non-expert dental settings. Case reports of successful application of behavioural therapies, including hypnotherapy, also exist.

Secondary headaches

Nocturnal or morning headache can occasionally be a symptom of more sinister underlying pathologies. Of these, the most pertinent to consider when assessing patients with prominent complaints of sleep-related or morning headache include:

- Hypertension (blood pressure surges in REM sleep; undiagnosed phaeochromocytomas)
- Recurrent nocturnal/morning hypoglycaemia in type 1 diabetes
- Metabolic disorders (including occult carbon monoxide poisoning)
- Vascular causes:
  - Reversible cerebral vasoconstriction syndrome:
    - Series of recurrent thunderclap headaches, which can be nocturnal
    - Usually transient, lasting 3 weeks
    - Can be complicated by stroke
    - More common in middle-aged women; SSRI and nasal decongestant use
  - Subarachnoid haemorrhage
- Ophthalmic causes, e.g. acute angle glaucoma—typically presents in early morning hours.

Postural effects also need to be considered. Headache consistently worsened by recumbency raises the possibility of increased intracranial pressure. Conversely, 'orthostatic' headache consistently improved by flat bed rest, and worsened by erect posture, are strongly suggestive of low CSF pressure (intracranial hypotension), caused either as a sequel of spinal interventions, or occurring spontaneously.

Further reading

Evers S (Ed). Special issue on headache and sleep. Cephalalgia. 2014;34(10):723–24.
Holle D, Naegel S, Obermann M. Hypnic headache. Cephalalgia. 2013;33(16):1349–57.
Nesbitt AD, Goadsby PJ. Cluster headache. BMJ. 2012;344:e2407.

Sleep and epilepsy

Sofia Eriksson

Introduction

There is a complex relationship between sleep and epilepsy. Some epileptic seizures mainly occur during sleep and may represent a differential diagnostic challenge from parasomnias, and vice versa. Epilepsy may be exacerbated by sleep deprivation and sleep disorders disrupting sleep may therefore worsen epilepsy. Finally, epilepsy and antiseizure medications may aggravate some sleep disorders.

Circadian influence on cortical excitability and distribution of seizures

The propensity of epileptic seizures to occur in temporal patterns has been known since the Babylonians, and Gowers, in the late nineteenth century, classified seizures as diurnal, nocturnal, or diffuse.

The tendency for seizures to occur during a specific time of day appears to be at least partly influenced by seizure onset zone, where frontal lobe seizures occur predominantly during sleep. Temporal lobe seizures happen mostly in wakefulness in a bimodal distribution, with a primary peak in the late afternoon and a secondary peak in the morning. Epileptic seizures can occur at any stage of NREM sleep but are more frequent during changes between sleep stages and lighter stages than deep sleep. Seizures rarely occur during REM sleep.

During sleep, there is progressive synchronization within the thalamocortical network that enables the generation of NREM sleep oscillations such as slow waves and sleep spindles. Similar circuits are thought to be involved in the generation of spike-wave discharges in generalized epilepsies. Interictal epileptiform discharges peak during normal sleep hours, regardless of location of the seizure onset zone. It therefore seems, that while interictal epileptiform discharge activation is principally favoured by sleep, the transition from interictal to ictal state is modulated by circadian factors related to the location of the epileptic network or epilepsy type.

Sleep deprivation is a common trigger to epileptic seizures. Studies using transcranial magnetic stimulation have demonstrated that cortical excitability increases with time awake which also appears to vary according to epilepsy syndrome, with bilateral changes seen in generalized epilepsy but only ipsilateral changes in focal epilepsy. Excitability is also modulated by circadian phase, such that cortical excitability is lower in the evening hours. It would therefore appear that the circadian timing system, sleep homeostasis (i.e. the duration of wakefulness and sleep), as well as vigilance states all contribute to the cortical inhibitory and excitatory balance.

Sleep-related epilepsy

Clinical features and epidemiology

Three main types of seizures occurring from sleep were described in the 1990s:

- Paroxysmal arousals:
  - Abrupt arousal from sleep
  - Highly stereotyped (similar each time) motor activity and/or vocalization
  - Dystonic posturing of the limbs or grimacing/fearful facial expressions are commonly seen
  - Often very brief, a matter of seconds, and may be under-reported, occurring without awareness
- Nocturnal paroxysmal dystonia:
  - Often beginning with a paroxysmal arousal, but followed by more complex movements
  - May be simple dystonic posturing of the limbs, but are often bizarre, such as rhythmic rocking or twisting movements of the trunk or pelvis. Vocalizations are also common
  - Events are usually brief, <2 minutes, sometimes much shorter, with abrupt offset
- Episodic nocturnal wanderings:
  - Usually occurring after an event as described previously, with exiting the bed and walking around in an agitated manner, screaming or other vocalizations, ranging from simple moaning or grunting, to comprehensible words
  - May exhibit more complex automatisms, which may appear semi-purposeful, such as cycling, running, or kicking.

The term nocturnal frontal lobe epilepsy was previously commonly used. Since the attacks are associated with sleep rather than time of day, and the seizures may arise from extrafrontal brain regions, it was recently recommended to change the name to sleep-related hypermotor epilepsy (SHE).

The prevalence of SHE is 1.8–1.9 per 100,000 in the adult population. The aetiology of SHE may be genetic or due to structural pathology, but remains unknown in many cases.

Diagnostic testing

Diagnostic testing includes:

- MRI brain imaging—performed to explore potential underlying causes for epilepsy. Any cerebral lesion, such as tumour, stroke, congenital vascular malformation, or cortical dysplasia, may cause epileptic seizures
- Interictal EEG (recording between attacks) is normal in the majority of patients with SHE. Interictal epileptiform discharges are seen in 45% of sleep EEG and 33% of wake EEG
- Ictal EEG—even during events, the EEG is often normal or obscured by muscle artefacts.

To facilitate differential diagnosis between epilepsy and parasomnias, particularly NREM parasomnias, a number of scales and scores have been developed, mainly based on clinical characteristics of events. The sensitivity and specificity of these scales has not been established and they are rarely used in everyday clinical practice. There are some clinical features that may help in differentiating nocturnal events, as outlined in ➔ Table 17.1, p. 166; e.g. stereotypy and dystonic posturing are more common features in seizures, while waxing and waning, prolonged duration, and indistinct offset are more common in parasomnias.

Semiology—clinical features witnessed—of sleep-related events, as recorded on video, can play a key role in distinguishing epileptic seizures from sleep disorders, predominantly parasomnias. Home video can provide valuable data and is recommended.

Three diagnostic levels of SHE have been suggested:

- Witnessed (possible) SHE: the semiological aspects of SHE hypermotor seizures, as provided by an eyewitness, and data from a good clinical history are sufficient to make the diagnosis of witnessed (possible) SHE
- Video-documented (clinical) SHE: clinically diagnosed SHE requires audio-video documentation of hypermotor events. At least one (but preferably two) entire events should be documented (confirmed to be typical by witness), including the onset, the evolution, and offset of the attacks
- Video-EEG-documented (confirmed) SHE: this requires video-EEG documentation of the events. SHE is confirmed when hypermotor seizures are recorded during sleep, associated with a clear-cut epileptic discharge or with interictal epileptiform abnormalities.

Sleep disorders exacerbating epilepsy

EDS or sleep complaints are common in patients with epilepsy and are often attributed to antiseizure medication. It is, however, important to consider concomitant sleep disorders that might cause EDS and may also worsen seizure control:

- OSA seems to be more common in patients with epilepsy than in the general population and may be related to the severity of epilepsy. The risk factors for OSA are, however, the same as in the general population (male sex, obesity, older age):
  - May fragment sleep as well as cause sleep deprivation, both of which may have a detrimental effect on seizure control
  - Should be considered in epilepsy patients who lose seizure control, particularly if there are risk factors for OSA
  - Improvement of seizure control has been seen after successful treatment of OSA
  - Treating SDB should be considered independently of its severity in epilepsy patients who are not seizure free
- RLS and PLMS – incidences in patients with epilepsy are not known but the disorders should be considered in patients with daytime somnolence:
  - If associated with sleep fragmentation, RLS and PLMS should be treated
  - Choice of antiseizure drugs (such as pregabalin or gabapentin) to treat RLS/PLMD may be preferable in patients with sleep-related epilepsy
- Insomnia is commonly reported in patients with epilepsy:
  - CBT should be considered the first-line treatment choice of chronic insomnia in patients with epilepsy, as with patients without epilepsy. However, caution should be adopted in using sleep restriction/compression as part of CBT as it may cause sleep deprivation, potentially triggering seizures
  - Pharmacological treatment may be used in treating insomnia in epilepsy patients, provided that utilized drugs do not interfere with seizure threshold.

Epilepsy and antiseizure treatment exacerbating sleep disorders

Seizures and frequent interictal epileptiform discharges can disrupt sleep architecture, causing more unstable sleep. Reduced amount of REM sleep has been seen after seizures.

Antiseizure medications have different effects on sleep (summarized in Table 25.1) and some also have different long- and short-term effects:

- Antiseizure medications may worsen OSA by reducing respiratory drive and upper airway tone (e.g. benzodiazepines and phenobarbitone) or contributing to weight gain (e.g. sodium valproate, pregabalin, and gabapentin)
- RLS and PMLS have been described in some patients treated with topiramate and zonisamide
- Insomnia is often reported in patients treated with lamotrigine. Changing dose regimens, taking a lower dose in the evening, or taking the evening dose earlier in the afternoon, may improve symptoms but this has not been evaluated in any formal studies.

Vagus nerve stimulation, a palliative procedure to reduce seizure frequency in patients with medically refractory epilepsy, has been shown to induce or worsen SDB in some patients, possibly via alterations of laryngeal motility.

Table 25.1 Anti-seizure medications and their influences on sleep

ASM	Effects on sleep in epilepsy								Effects on sleep disorders	
	SE/TST	SL	WASO	N1	N2	N3	REM	Arousals	Improvement	Worsening
Phenobarbital	↑	↓	–	–	↑	–	↓	↓	Insomnia	OSA
Phenytoin	–	↓	–	↑	↑	↓/↑	–/↓	–	None	None
Carbamazepine	–	–	–	–	–	↑	↑	↑	RLS	NONE
Valproate	–	–	–	↑	↓	–	–	–	None	OSA*
Gabapentin	–	–	–	–/↑	–	↑	↑	↓	RLS	OSA*
Lamotrigine	–	–	–	–	↑/–	↓/–	↑/–	–	None	Insomnia
Topiramate	–	–/↓	–	–	–	–	–	–	OSA*	RLS PLMD†
Levetiracetam	–	–	–	–	↑	↑	–	–	None	None
Pregabalin	↑	–	–	↓	–	↑	–	–	RLS	OSA*
Zonisamide	–	–	–	–	–	–	–	–	OSA*	RLS
Lacosamide	–	–	–	–	–	–	–	↑	None	None
Eslicarbazepine	–	–	–	–	–	↑	–	–	None	None
Perampanel	–	–	↓	–	–	–	–	–	Insomnia RLS	None

*Due to weight change. †Few case reports.

–, No change; ↑, increase; ↓, decrease; OSA, obstructive sleep apnoea; PLMD, periodic limb movement disorder; REM, rapid eye movement; RLS, restless leg syndrome; SE sleep efficiency; SL sleep latency; TST total sleep time; WASO wakefulness after sleep onset.

Management

Sleep-related epilepsies should be treated with antiseizure medication. In the early descriptions of nocturnal frontal lobe epilepsy, carbamazepine was often suggested as an effective first-line treatment. Other antiseizure medications may be as effective, and first-line choice should be tailored according to individual patient characteristics.

Conclusion

There is a close relationship between sleep and epilepsy. Correctly diagnosing paroxysmal nocturnal events remains a challenge. Sleep disorders are common in patients with epilepsy and it is important for clinicians to ask about sleep and symptoms of sleep disorders and consider alternative causes to loss of seizure control or excessive daytime somnolence than antiseizure medication. Identification and treatment of concomitant sleep disorders in epilepsy is important for optimal patient care.

Further reading

Derry CP, Harvey AS, Walker MC, et al. NREM arousal parasomnias and their distinction from nocturnal frontal lobe epilepsy: a video EEG analysis. Sleep 2009;32(12):1637–44.

Khan S, Nobili L, Khatami R, et al. Circadian rhythm and epilepsy. Lancet Neurol. 2018;17(12):1098–108.

Tinuper P, Bisulli F, Cross JH, et al. Definition and diagnostic criteria of sleep-related hypermotor epilepsy. Neurology. 2016;86(19):1834–42.

Sleep and pain

Alexander D. Nesbitt

Introduction

Chronic pain affects 10% of the population, and 50–75% of people with chronic pain report sleep difficulties. Pain disrupts sleep continuity and quality via many different mechanisms, and conversely, poor sleep, short sleep, and prolonged sleep can amplify chronic pain, in an often bidirectional relationship.

These interactions relate to numerous disorders causing chronic pain, and are not necessarily specific to any particular one. Causes of chronic pain, in which a majority of sufferers commonly report poor sleep, include:

- Abdominal pain (irritable bowel syndrome, dyspepsia, bladder disorders)
- Cancer pain (direct invasion, hypercalcaemia)
- Rheumatological pain (arthritis, fibromyalgia)
- Neuropathic pain (burns, neuropathy)
- Post-traumatic pain
- Orofacial and dental pain.

Sleep-related symptoms can include insomnia, EDS, RLS, snoring, and, more unusually, abnormal sleep behaviours. Sleep behavioural ('hygiene') practices are often poor.

Drugs influencing sleep

Use of prescribed medication can frequently cause significant sleep disturbances. In the context of pain, this includes:

- Opioids:
  - EDS
  - SDB
- Antidepressants:
  - Insomnia in alerting medications
  - REM disruption
  - RLS and PLMD
- Non-steroidal anti-inflammatory drugs:
  - Melatonin suppression
  - Gastro-oesophageal reflux.

Coexisting symptoms complicating sleep

Common coexisting symptoms in patients with chronic pain, many of which also impact sleep, include:

- Often overwhelming fatigue (more so than EDS)
- Mood disturbances (including MDD)
- Anxiety
- Often vague cognitive and memory complaints
- Lack of exercise leading to autonomic deconditioning (including orthostatic symptoms, sweating)
- Nightmares may also be more frequent
- Substance dependency is also a common problem, in terms of prescription medications (opioids, benzodiazepines), alcohol, and illicit drug use (particularly cannabis).

Sleep complicating pain

Mechanisms involved in this relationship may include:
- SWS loss probably promotes nociception more than REM loss
- There may be circadian changes in pain amplitude (pain often worse in morning)
- Sleep fragmentation increases pro-inflammatory cytokines (interleukin-6, tumour necrosis factor-alpha)
- Sleep fragmentation alters hypothalamic–pituitary stress responses
- There may be long-term plastic changes in higher-order pain modulation networks
- Cognitive perception of pain may be worsened by sleep disruption.

Objective PSG findings are not specific for chronic pain, and PSG should only be considered if there is a strong suspicion of additional primary sleep pathologies. Changes seen include:
- Poor sleep efficiency
- Increased sleep latency
- Increased wake after sleep onset
- Increase in N1, N2, and decrease in N3
- Higher arousal index
- Alpha intrusions in SWS (alpha-delta)
- Phasic arousal changes (cyclic alternating pattern).

Sleep pathology may be present, and likely multifactorial in origin. Commonly identified problems include:
- SDB (immobility, weight gain, opioid use)
  - OSA
  - CSA (sleep-onset CSA, opioid use)
- Periodic limb movements (antidepressant use)
- Bruxism
- Occasionally, NREM arousal parasomnias in predisposed individuals.

Possible management options

A multidimensional approach to treatment is often the most effective strategy. While improvements can be made, these are often small, but may have an overall cumulative effect. Strategies can include:

- Behavioural sleep improvements:
  - Environment controls (optimizing pillow, mattress, and positioning comfort)
  - Usual sleep advice, including removal of devices, TV, and pets from bedroom
  - Adequate daylight exposure
  - Dim evening environment
  - Not resting in bed, and avoiding daytime naps
- Non-pharmacological strategies:
  - Hot/cold applications
  - Physiotherapy
  - Massages
  - Progressive muscle relaxation and mentalization-based techniques
  - Mindfulness
  - Transcutaneous electrical nerve stimulation machines
  - There may be a role for CBT-I in some patients
- Pharmacological strategies:
  - Acute analgesia (paracetamol probably preferable in evenings)
  - Local analgesia (lidocaine patches, capsaicin creams)
  - Muscle relaxants (consider baclofen in some)
  - Short-term hypnotic use (Z drugs, benzodiazepines)
  - Chronobiotics (low-dose melatonin)
  - Sleep-promoting neuropathic agents:
    - Amitriptyline or nortriptyline
    - Gabapentin
    - Pregabalin
  - Sleep-promoting antidepressants:
    - Trazodone (beware—may worsen chronic migraine)
    - Mirtazapine
    - Doxepin
    - Dosulepin.

Where possible, long-term use of opioids should be avoided, and opioids slowly withdrawn and substituted with suggestions included previously.

It is also important to try and identify and treat comorbidities, including active depression and anxiety (with psychological therapies, and drugs which may promote sleep (see earlier)), as well as fatigue (graded exercise therapy).

Further reading

Choy EH. The role of sleep in pain and fibromyalgia. Nat Rev Rheumatol. 2015;11(9):513–20.

Tang NK, Lereya ST, Boulton H, et al. Nonpharmacological treatments of insomnia for long-term painful conditions: a systematic review and meta-analysis of patient-reported outcomes in randomized controlled trials. Sleep. 2015;38(11):1751–64.

Tang NK, Wright KJ, Salkovskis PM. Prevalence and correlates of clinical insomnia co-occurring with chronic back pain. J Sleep Res. 2007;16(1):85–95.

Sleep and psychiatric disorders

Ivana Rosenzweig and *Ricardo S. Osorio*

Introduction

Sleep disturbance affects 50–80% of all patients with psychiatric disorders. Sleep has a vital role in immune, metabolic, and central nervous system regeneration and maintenance, in memory consolidation, and affect regulation. SWS and REM sleep have been of significant interest to neurologists, psychiatrists, and psychologists—SWS because of its putative role in brain repair, detoxification, homeostatic maintenance, and in cognitive function, and REM sleep because of its suggested involvement in memory, neurodevelopment, and emotional regulation. To date, little is known about the consequences of disrupted sleep and sleep deprivation in psychiatric disorders. Moreover, in clinical practice, sleep disturbance is still often regarded as an epiphenomenon of the primary psychiatric disorder.

Sleep disorders increase the risk of developing episodes of psychiatric disorders. Patients with OSA have a 1.8-fold increased risk of developing depression and those with depression have a 1.6-fold increased risk for OSA. Also, insomnia, defined as difficulty initiating or maintaining sleep resulting in daytime consequences, is common among psychiatric disorders. Several other potential comorbid sleep disorders, including OSA, RLS, PLMD, and RBD are known to modulate psychiatric symptom expression.

It is increasingly recognized that sleep and psychiatric disorders may share a bidirectional relationship. Therefore, concurrent and aggressive management of sleep should be a pivotal part of the clinical management in all psychiatric disorders.

Clinical considerations

The presence of disturbed sleep either forms an essential part of, or at the minimum is listed as one of the recognized pivotal symptoms for, several major psychiatric disorders in the *Diagnostic and Statistical Manual of Mental Disorders* and the International Classification of Diseases. This includes the diagnostic criteria for major depressive disorder (MDD), BPAD, generalized anxiety disorder (GAD), PTSD, and schizophrenia.

Major depressive disorder

Major depression affects an estimated 10–25% of women and 5–12% of men. It has an onset in early adulthood. Sleep disturbances are highly prevalent in patients with depression (90%) and many sleep disorders (e.g. OSA, narcolepsy, insomnia) are associated with increased risk of developing MDD.

Subjective sleep complaints
- Difficulty falling asleep (initial insomnia)
- Frequent nocturnal awakenings
- Early morning awakening
- Decreased or increased total sleep
- Insufficient sleep quality
- Nightmares.

Practical clinical considerations
- Increased risk (up to ten times) in patients with significant insomnia or hypersomnia
- About 20–44% of patients with MDD continue to suffer residual sleep issues despite the adequate administration of pharmacotherapy (e.g. antidepressants) and/or talking therapy (e.g. CBT)
- Residual insomnia is associated with an increased risk of relapse and an increased risk of residual cognitive deficits
- MDD patients with poor sleep have slower treatment response and lower remission rates than those without sleep disturbance
- Poor sleep is independently correlated with poorer quality of life
- Inter-episodic persistence of subjective sleep disruption predicts increased severity and recurrence of MDD
- Hypersomnia is the main symptom in some depressive disorders, such as seasonal affective depression and depression with atypical features, or in depressive episodes in BPAD.

Polysomnographic findings
The significance of the alterations in sleep and sleep stages is of uncertain and limited clinical utility, as they are not specific to those with MDD. However, PSG findings in MDD include:
- REM sleep: shortened latency to the onset of REM sleep (REM latency), increased number of eye movements per minute of REM sleep (REM density); increased percentage of the night that meets scoring criteria for REM sleep; a longer duration of the first REM period
- SWS deficit: decreased amount of SWS
- Shortened REM latency and reduced SWS are the most significant *trait* markers
- Increased REM density and sleep disturbance are the *state* markers most evident during acute episodes.

Sleep deprivation
- Total, partial, and a chronic REM sleep deprivation may have a profound effect on individuals with mood disorders; especially those with a pronounced diurnal pattern of illness
- A night of total sleep deprivation has been reported to have robust antidepressant effects that peak by the afternoon
- Clinical utility of sleep deprivation as a treatment is limited, and the benefits generally disappear when the treated patient sleeps again, even if the period of sleep is short.

Risk factor for suicide
- Sleep disturbance leads to significantly increased risk of suicidal ideation, suicide attempts, and completed suicide in all age groups
- The clinical management plan in MDD should include careful monitoring of sleep and it should specify its management as an important means of preventing suicide in those with MDD.

Bipolar affective disorder

In contrast to MDD, BPAD affects ~1% of the population and it has no sex predilection. Sleep deprivation tends to exacerbate symptoms in those with BPAD, predisposing individuals to develop manic episodes. The mechanisms by which sleep loss might predispose patients with BPAD to develop mania are not known. However, notably, most antimanic therapies to date have significant sleep-enhancing effects and for the manic or hypomanic phase of BPAD, the diagnostic criteria include almost a pathognomonic decreased need for sleep, during which patients do not experience significant impairment in function. It has also been suggested that the transition from euthymia or depression to the manic stage occurs during sleep.

Subjective sleep complaints
- Reduced total sleep time (diagnostic confusion with insomnia)
- A subjective sensation of a decreased need for sleep with no significant daytime functional deficits
- Conversely, hypersomnia is the most common complaint during the depressed phase and it occurs more frequently in those with BPAD than in patients with MD
- No objective evidence of clinically significant daytime sleepiness in patients using the MSLT.

Polysomnographic findings
- Comparable to sleep changes reported in MDD
- Lithium, used for the treatment of patients with BPAD, may cause or exacerbate RLS; increases SWS, suppresses REM sleep, and increases latency

Generalized anxiety and other anxiety disorders

Lifetime prevalence of chronic anxiety and excessive, pervasive worry (GAD) is ~6%. Sleep disturbance is a core feature of GAD (difficulty falling or staying asleep), affecting over half of patients.

Insomnia may double the risk for the subsequent development of anxiety disorders. Studies support the clinical importance of targeted insomnia therapy in GAD and other anxiety patients. It is less clear whether the treatment of insomnia might impact GAD outcome.

Subjective sleep complaints
- Panic attacks evolving from sleep may result in insomnia because sleep may become regarded as an anxiogenic state
- Of patients with panic disorder, 68% identify problems falling asleep and 77% report difficulties maintaining adequate sleep
- Between 44% and 71% of patients with panic disorder experience sleep panic attacks, with 18–45% of panic attacks arising from sleep.

Practical clinical considerations
- Treatment for these conditions is commonly prolonged
- Benzodiazepines (e.g. clonazepam) are extensively used and the available evidence suggests that the anxiolytic effects persist and are not associated with dosage escalation
- SSRIs and the dual reuptake inhibitors (SNRIs, e.g. venlafaxine) are efficacious, and unlike benzodiazepines they also treat comorbid depression
- Tricyclic antidepressants and antihistamines may also be helpful
- In a large cross-sectional study, 61% of panic disorder patients and 44% of patients with GAD were shown to have insomnia
- RLS is underdiagnosed in patients with anxiety disorders
- RLS and anxiety disorders, especially panic disorder, highly overlap, possibly due to a common dopaminergic abnormality
- Antidepressant use is linked to RLS, including the tricyclics and SSRIs, venlafaxine, and, particularly, mirtazapine
- Bupropion is neutral for RLS symptoms and could be helpful for RLS because of its dopaminergic activity
- The role of pregabalin, gabapentin, and tiagabine in the treatment of comorbid RLS/insomnia and psychiatric disorders (especially anxiety and mood disorders) is increasingly being explored
- Pregabalin is used off-label by sleep physicians. It is licensed in the UK for GAD, and it is used as an off-label treatment for periodic limb movements, middle insomnia, and sleep fragmentation; some studies suggest that it may also be effective in the adjunctive treatment of acute mania, depression, and in maintenance of refractory BPAD
- CBT is highly effective in treating GAD and insomnia, and is highly recommended in older adults, where benzodiazepines may be relatively contraindicated due to concerns about adverse effects.

Polysomnographic findings
- Increased sleep onset latency, a greater number of arousals, and increased wake time during the night
- No marked alterations in REM latency or its duration
- Nocturnal panic attacks typically occur at the transition between stages 2 and 3 of NREM sleep and are distinct from night terrors and other parasomnias, as well as from panic attacks occurring after nocturnal awakening.

Post-traumatic stress disorder

PTSD is characterized by the unwanted, recurrent re-experiencing of a previous profoundly disturbing, life-threatening episode, leading to functional impairment, avoidance, and hyperarousal symptoms. Lifetime prevalence is around 8% and it is twice as prevalent in women. Alcohol and substance abuse or dependence are common, as are sleep disorders (e.g. OSA, parasomnias, insomnia) and other comorbid psychiatric disorders (MDD, panic disorder). It has been reported that the severity of sleep complaints mediates the relationship between PTSD and functional disability. Effective treatment of PTSD has to encompass all comorbid clinical entities.

Subjective sleep complaints

- Distressing dreams and nightmares (viewed as re-experiencing phenomena)
- Insomnia, with difficulties falling or staying asleep
- Patients with comorbid PTSD and OSA may not report the typical daytime somnolence as this may be masked by heightened anxiety; instead, they may report fatigue or tiredness.

Practical clinical considerations

- Nightmares occur in up to 96% of PTSD patients, predominantly emerging from REM sleep
- Patients exposed to trauma who later develop PTSD report dream mentation that to a certain degree replicates the traumatic event
- Several non-pharmacological measures have been shown to be beneficial for nightmares, including exposure, relaxation, and rescripting therapy, sleep dynamic therapy, hypnosis, imagery rehearsal therapy, and CBT, either alone or in combination
- Eye movement desensitization and reprocessing (EMDR) may also help with sleep efficiency in PTSD
- OSA is highly prevalent in PTSD patients and the treatment of underlying OSA with CPAP may significantly improve nightmares and insomnia symptoms
- SSRIs (e.g. sertraline and paroxetine) and to a lesser extent tricyclic antidepressants and monoamine oxidase inhibitors may be useful
- Prazosin (alpha-1 adrenergic receptor antagonist) and the adjunctive of mono-therapeutic use of atypical antipsychotics (e.g. quetiapine, olanzapine, risperidone) show early promising beneficial dual effects.

Polysomnographic findings

- Diminished total sleep time
- An elevation in the time spent awake after initially falling asleep
- An association between an increase in wake time after sleep onset and nightmares
- REM sleep alterations, including an increase in REM density (eye movements per minute of REM sleep) has been reported.

Schizophrenia

Schizophrenia has a lifetime prevalence of 0.5–1%. It is a debilitating neurodevelopmental disorder, with onset commonly in late adolescence. Characterized by psychotic symptoms comprising delusions and/or hallucinations, disorganization of speech and/or behaviour, and deficits in functional capacity. Impairment in cognitive and executive function often occur. Sleep and circadian rhythm disorders, while not a core symptom of schizophrenia, are nonetheless frequently reported. Systematic epidemiological data on the prevalence of sleep disturbances in this population do not exist; however, increases in the prevalence of OSA (15%), PLMS, and insomnia have been documented. Severe insomnia can be a prodromal symptom to psychotic decompensation and/or relapse to psychosis following antipsychotic discontinuation.

Subjective sleep complaints
- Severe sleep disturbance is common prior to the development of episodes of acute psychosis, and it may constitute an important part of a relapse
- Even among clinically stable and medicated patients, early and middle insomnia are common
- Patients commonly complain about poor sleep quality, restlessness, agitation, and nightmares.

Practical clinical considerations
- Antipsychotic treatment in schizophrenia may lead to excessive daytime sedation, which can facilitate a reversal of the sleep–wake cycle and paradoxically exacerbate insomnia
- Metabolic dysregulation is common and it may lead to obesity and the increased risk of developing OSA
- OSA is commonly unrecognized in this patient group and it can contribute to exacerbation of neuropsychiatric symptoms, including aggressive behaviours. There are anecdotal reports of the beneficial effect of CPAP treatment in patients with comorbid OSA and schizophrenia
- The hypnagogic and hypnopompic hallucinations of narcolepsy can be misdiagnosed as psychotic symptoms of schizophrenia. This has significant treatment implications, as stimulant therapy may ameliorate hypnagogic and hypnopompic hallucinations but can exacerbate schizophrenia:
  - Narcoleptic hallucinations: often characterized by a multimodal perceptual experience including visual, auditory, and tactile elements
  - Frank schizophrenic hallucinations: unimodal and frequently auditory, accompanied by delusional symptoms and limited insight.

Polysomnographic findings
- Increased latency to sleep onset
- Increased wake time during the night
- Decreased total sleep time
- Decreased latency to the onset of REM sleep
- Decreased sleep spindle density and amplitude
- Decreased amount of SWS, and a decrease in the amplitude of EEG slow waves during non-REM sleep

- *Positive symptoms* such as delusions, hallucinations, and disorganized thought have been correlated with shorter REM latency, longer sleep onset latency, and diminished sleep efficiency
- *Negative symptoms* (e.g. affective flattening, avolition, alogia, attention problems) severity has been found to be correlated with lower non-REM sleep EEG slow-wave amplitude and shorter REM onset latency
- A greater percentage of the night spent in REM sleep and greater REM density have been correlated with an increased risk of suicidal ideation in schizophrenia.

The clinical significance and pathophysiological implications of these findings remain uncertain as the PSG alterations described are not solely specific to schizophrenia and the findings have not been consistently found across studies.

Substance abuse

Substance abuse and dependency is common. Substances with a high abuse liability have a profound effect on sleep. Sleep difficulties including insomnia increase the risk of substance abuse.

Practical clinical considerations

Alcoholism

Disruption of the circadian sleep–wake rhythm and insomnia (in 36–72%) are common:

- Sleep disturbance and a relative increase in REM sleep may persist for several years of abstinence from alcohol
- The link between disturbed sleep during abstinence and relapse to drinking has been identified in several studies
- Sleep disturbance originates from a rebound of wakefulness following the initial sedation and the hypnotic effect by alcohol
- Alcohol suppresses REM sleep and relatively increases the amount of non-REM sleep, but those effects are short-lived and subsequent sleep disruption and increased REM activity occur, leading to middle insomnia and nightmares. This problem is escalated when tolerance develops to the hypnotic effects with repeated use
- Alcohol use may also exacerbate several other sleep disorders, including OSA, PLMD, and RLS, as well as parasomnias such as sleepwalking and RBD
- OSA and snoring are worsened by alcohol, even after a single drink
- PLMD and RLS prevalence increases two- to threefold in patients having two or more drinks per day
- Exacerbation of parasomnias, such as sleepwalking, may also have distinct forensic implications, including 'sexsomnia', a potentially violent parasomnia where sexual behaviours are enacted in sleep
- Benzodiazepines and Z drugs (e.g. zopiclone, zolpidem, and zaleplon) for the treatment of insomnia are avoided because of their abuse potential in abstinent alcoholics
- Medications shown to improve sleep disturbances in this population include trazodone, carbamazepine, acamprosate, pregabalin, and gabapentin.

Cannabis (tetrahydrocannabinol)
- Effects can be variable because it contains numerous compounds, some with sedative effects and others with wakefulness-promoting properties such as cannabidiol
- Decreased REM sleep and its density are reported in marijuana users
- *Nabilone*, a synthetic cannabinoid, has been used with some success in the treatment of PTSD nightmares
- Tetrahydrocannabinol withdrawal has been associated with sleep disturbances, with disturbing dreams most consistently reported; withdrawal symptoms begin 2–3 days after the last use and they can persist up to 7 weeks.

Opioids
- High abuse liability with disruptive effect on sleep continuity and sleep architecture
- Acute administration causes reductions in total sleep time, REM sleep, and SWS
- In opioid withdrawal, insomnia frequently occurs, with reduced SWS and markedly diminished REM sleep
- Although not the first line of treatment, opioids improve RLS; contraindicated in OSA
- Several studies report a high prevalence of central and complex apnoea in patients on methadone maintenance treatment; CPAP of servo-ventilation treatment shows mixed success
- In chronic heroin users, maximal REM and SWS suppression occurs 2–3 days into abstinence, and some suppression persists for 5–7 days into abstinence
- In methadone users, REM and SWS rebound occurs 13–22 weeks after methadone withdrawal and can lead to late stage behavioural changes.

Cocaine
- Acute effects of cocaine upon sleep resemble those of other psychostimulants such as amphetamine. A longer sleep latency, reduced total sleep time, and suppression of REM sleep are noted
- During acute cocaine withdrawal, total sleep time is significantly reduced resembling that of untreated chronic insomniacs; sleep onset latency is prolonged and sleep efficiency is decreased with an increase in REM sleep percentage, and reduced REM latency also observed (consistent with the subjective withdrawal symptom of increased dreaming)
- Cognitive performance significantly deteriorates during subacute cocaine withdrawal (around day 10); however, of note is that this is commonly not recognized by patients and that they subjectively report an improvement in sleep during subacute withdrawal, an exact opposite of the distorted sleep perception in primary insomniacs, who underestimate their sleep quality. It has been suggested that this paradox might be due to an increase in delta spectral power which is associated with better self-reports of sleep quality.

In patients whose comorbid mood and sleep disorders are unrecognized and hence untreated, drug-seeking behaviour may be maintained by the substance's mood altering and euphorigenic effects, as well as its therapeutic effects (self-medication) for any comorbid sleep or mood disorder.

Treatment considerations in psychiatric patients

Treatments for psychiatric disorders commonly modify sleep architecture, and vice versa, treatments for sleep disorders may increase the risks for psychiatric disorders.

Effects of drugs on sleep

Antidepressants
- Used off-label for the treatment of insomnia and sleep fragmentation; prescribed in lower doses than when used to treat MDD
- Trazodone, mirtazapine, amitriptyline, and doxepin are among the most frequent medications used by sleep physicians
- However, data from placebo-controlled trials exist only for doxepin and trimipramines
- Monoamine oxidase inhibitors, tricyclic antidepressants, electroconvulsive therapy, SSRIs, and SNRIs all suppress REM sleep
- Bupropion, nefazodone, mirtazapine, and trazodone have negligible effects on REM sleep and tend to increase the amount of SWS and the amplitude of EEG slow waves in non-REM sleep
- Acamprosate (a N-methyl-D-aspartic acid receptor antagonist and positive allosteric modulator of $GABA_A$ receptors), used in treatment of alcoholism, has been reported to decrease wake time after sleep onset and to cause a shortened REM latency.

Antipsychotics
- The mainstay of schizophrenia treatment; also used as adjunctive or monotherapy in MDD, BPAD, and anxiety disorders
- First-generation (typical) antipsychotics are primarily dopaminergic antagonists, with antihistaminergic and anticholinergic effects
- Second-generation (atypical) antipsychotics have the added effect of blocking serotonergic receptors and are associated with improvement of negative and cognitive symptoms
- Atypical antipsychotics differentially affect sleep architecture but are overall recognized to improve sleep efficiency; they tend to shorten sleep onset latency and supress REM sleep
- The central H_1 antihistaminergic effects of antipsychotics have significant sedating properties; this likely underlies some of their sleep-promoting and maintaining effect; prescribed in lower doses when used to treat sleep disorders
- The highest rates of sedation are reported with clozapine and chlorpromazine (60%), followed by risperidone and olanzapine (30%), and haloperidol (23%); the least sedation is reported with quetiapine and ziprasidone (16%) and aripiprazole (12%).

Common adverse effects on sleep
- Insomnia and sleep disturbance can be caused by bupropion, SSRIs, and venlafaxine
- Neuroleptics can cause or exacerbate PLMS and RLS due to their dopamine antagonism
- SSRIs, SNRIs, lithium, quetiapine, and mirtazapine, are frequently associated with RLS and PLMD

- Neuroleptics used in psychiatric disorders may lead to increased weight and may increase the risks of developing metabolic syndrome and OSA
- Historically, antidepressants were reported to trigger symptoms of RBD in up to 6% of patients. However, MDD and RBD are likely an early symptom of one of the underlying neurodegenerative synucleinopathies, including PD, DLB, and MSA and these drugs may simply unmask RBD rather than triggering it.

Further reading

Baglioni C, Nanovska S, Regen W, et al. Sleep and mental disorders: a meta-analysis of polysomnographic research. Psychol Bull. 2016;142(9):969–90.

Krystal AD. Psychiatric disorders and sleep. Neurol Clin. 2012;30(4):1389–413.

Schierenbeck T, Riemann D, Berger M, et al. Effect of illicit recreational drugs upon sleep: cocaine, ecstasy and marijuana. Sleep Med Rev. 2008;12(5):381–89.

Medications influencing sleep

Elaine Lyons and *Grainne d'Ancona*

Introduction

As we age, the nature of our sleep—in terms of architecture and duration—changes. But, in addition, the accrual of morbidities throughout life frequently gives rise to an increasing pharmacological burden, with polypharmacy a commonly encountered situation. Many medications have an under-recognized impact on sleep, through their effects on neurotransmitter function and alteration of sleep architecture, although often, the mechanism whereby a drug causes a disruption of sleep/wakefulness is not fully understood. In many cases, a simple amendment to the dose regimen may address the problem (e.g. changing the timing of doses), but in others, an alternative should be sought. In any patient with a sleep complaint, the drug history—both for prescribed and non-prescribed medications—should be carefully examined.

This chapter will briefly address the following:
- Drugs causing sleepiness
- Drugs causing insomnia
- Drugs used in the management of sleep disorders.

Drugs causing sleepiness

Several medicines are known to cause somnolence, and users should be advised of this (these medicines carry a mandatory warning on the need to avoid potentially hazardous activities while taking it, e.g. driving). Occasionally, patients will ascribe sleepiness to a drug without this being a recognized side effect and clinicians should be aware that, at toxic levels, some drugs (particularly those with a narrow therapeutic window) may cause drowsiness.

In some cases, sedation is a desirable side effect and tolerance to it may develop. Where it is troublesome, the medicine may be equally effective if administered at night, or a non-sedating alternative should be considered. Table 28.1 lists commonly prescribed medicines with sedating effects, and potential ways to minimize the impact of this. The list is not exhaustive, so always consult the product literature (e.g. ✎ https://www.medicines.org.uk/emc/ sections 4.7 and 4.8).

Table 28.1 Drugs known to cause sleepiness

Drug class	Proposed effect(s) on sleep	Assuaging effect
Antidepressants Tricyclic antidepressants, mirtazapine, trazodone	Suppresses REM sleep. Causes neurochemical imbalances directly (e.g. serotonin, dopamine, and noradrenaline (norepinephrine)) or indirectly. This neurochemical depletion over time can lead to fatigue. May disrupt the normal pattern of melatonin secretion. Some agents also have an antihistaminergic effect	Administer at night or switch to a less sedating antidepressant, e.g. an SSRI
Antihistamines E.g. chlorphenamine (chlorpheniramine)	Older agents cross the blood–brain barrier (BBB) and by disrupting normal histamine function around regulating sleep and wakefulness, cause drowsiness	Switch to a newer antihistamine that doesn't readily cross the BBB, e.g. loratadine, cetirizine
Antiemetics E.g. antihistamines, anticholinergics, phenothiazines, dopamine antagonists	Phenothiazines and dopamine antagonists suppress REM sleep, resulting in inefficient sleep and subsequent daytime drowsiness	Switch to alternative non-drowsy antiemetic, e.g. ondansetron

Drug class	Proposed effect(s) on sleep	Assuaging effect
Antipsychotics E.g. haloperidol	Antipsychotic medications vary in their sedative effect, primarily dependent on their affinity for histamine H_1 receptors. Drowsiness is usually dose related	May improve the quality of sleep, but consider an atypical antipsychotic e.g. quetiapine, risperidone, olanzapine, where sedation is often less frequent and less severe
Anticonvulsants Sodium valproate	May increase NREM sleep, and reduce REM sleep, and may result in daytime drowsiness	Take at bedtime as a prolonged-release preparation
Alpha-2-delta ligands (e.g. gabapentin or pregabalin)	Mechanism not fully understood, but may increase SWS	
Benzodiazepines E.g. diazepam **Non-benzodiazepine hypnotics** E.g. zopiclone, zolpidem	Binds $GABA_A$ receptor in the central nervous system	Take at bedtime and limit exposure
Opioids Morphine, oxycodone	Opioids binding to Mu2 in the central nervous system	Take at bedtime and limit exposure
Dopamine receptor agonists Rotigotine, ropinirole, pramipexole	Usually wake promoting but can affect sleep architecture, prolong sleep latency, and affect REM sleep in particular. Occasionally associated with sleep attacks	Consider alternative preparation
Leukotriene receptor antagonist E.g. montelukast		Take at night
5-HT$_1$ receptor agonist E.g. sumatriptan, rizatriptan		Drowsiness may be caused by the drug or migraine itself. It is usually mild–moderate and self-limiting due to short term use

Drugs causing insomnia

Several medicines prescribed for other indications can be alerting or disrupt night-time sleep, though not all patients report this effect. The effect of such medicines on sleep is best managed with morning dosing, minimizing the dose or changing to an alternative if necessary. Table 28.2 lists commonly prescribed medicines with potentially stimulating properties.

Table 28.2 Drugs known to cause insomnia

Drug class	Effect on sleep	Assuaging effect
Alpha-blockers E.g. doxazosin, tamsulosin	Decreased REM sleep	Take dose in the morning
Beta-blockers (lipophilic) E.g. metoprolol, propranolol	Reduces production and release of melatonin Reduces REM sleep	Take dose in the morning
Corticosteroids E.g. prednisolone	Reduces melatonin release	Take dose in the morning
Selective serotonin reuptake inhibitors (SSRIs) E.g. sertraline, fluoxetine, paroxetine	Suppresses REM sleep Increases sleep onset latency Increases number of awakenings and arousals, with overall significant decrease in sleep efficiency	Take dose in the morning Switch to alternative
Cholinesterase inhibitors E.g. donepezil, galantamine, rivastigmine	Increased REM sleep, abnormal dreams	Take dose in the morning Switch to shorter-acting preparation
Statins E.g. atorvastatin, rosuvastatin, simvastatin	Associated muscle pain can disrupt sleep pattern and cause abnormal dreams by restricting body's ability to rest	Reduce dose if possible; or switch to fibrate
Nicotine E.g. cigarette smoking or nicotine replacement therapy (NRT)	Increased difficulty in falling asleep, longer sleep latency, stimulant effect	Smoking cessation advice No smoking or NRT prior to bedtime
H$_1$ receptor antagonists E.g. cetirizine, fexofenadine, loratadine	Reduction in REM sleep Increases anxiety	Take in morning If possible, use as required only
Antimalarials E.g. atovaquone, mefloquine, chloroquine, proguanil, doxycycline		Take in the morning

Drug class	Effect on sleep	Assuaging effect
Caffeine E.g. Pro Plus®, some over-the-counter cold and flu remedies	Adenosine facilitates sleep and dilates the blood vessels. Caffeine is an adenosine receptor antagonist	Avoid after midday
Stimulants E.g. dexamfetamine, methylphenidate, modafinil	Increased difficulty in falling asleep, prolongs sleep onset, and overall shorter duration of sleep	Minimize the dose and take before 2 pm
Thyroid hormones E.g. thyroxine		Take in the morning

Drugs used in sleep disorders

The commonest sleep disorders in which prescribing is the norm are RLS/PLMD, RBD, non-REM parasomnias, and narcolepsy. Tables 28.3–28.6 include medicines that may be used to treat these disorders. Many are unlicensed for the indication, so always refer to manufacturers' and local guidance on their availability and use. The following tables are not a comprehensive list, and other agents may be used by specialist sleep physicians in appropriate circumstances.

Table 28.3 Drug used in narcolepsy

Starting dose	Maximum recommended dose	Time to therapeutic effect	Half-life
Modafinil			
100 mg daily (no later than 3 pm)	400 mg daily (divided doses and no later than 3 pm)	2–4 hours	15 hours
Methylphenidate ⚠ **U** 📈			
Extended-release XL 18 mg in the morning	108 mg every morning (divided doses and no later than 2 pm)	1–2 hours	3.5 hours
Instant release 10 mg (divided doses and no later than 2 pm)	60 mg daily in divided doses—no later than 2 pm	1–2 hours	2 hours
Dexamfetamine ⚠ **U** 📈			
10 mg daily (divided doses)—no later than 2 pm	60 mg daily (divided doses)—no later than 2 pm	1.5 hours	10 hours
Sodium oxybate ⚠ **(licensed for type 1 narcolepsy)**			
2.25. twice daily (first dose at bedtime, second dose 3 hours later)	4.5. twice daily (first dose at bedtime, second dose 3 hours later)	0.5–1 hour	6–8 hours
Pitolisant 📈			
9 mg in the morning	36 mg in the morning	3 hours	10–12 hours

Symbol	**Meaning**
📈	This medicinal product is subject to additional monitoring
U	Unlicensed
⚠	Controlled drug (requirements vary depending on schedule. Available at: https://www.gov.uk/government/publications/controlled-drugs-list--2/list-of-most-commonly-encountered-drugs-currently-controlled-under-the-misuse-of-drugs-legislation)

Table 28.4 Drugs used in restless legs syndrome/periodic limb movement disorder

Starting dose (at night)	Maximum recommended dosing (at night)	Time to therapeutic effect	Half-life
Ropinirole			
0.25 mg	4 mg	4–10 days	6 hours
Pramipexole			
0.088 mg	0.54 mg	4–10 days	8–12 hours
Rotigotine patch			
1 mg	3 mg	1 week	5–7 hours
Gabapentin ⚠ **U**			
300 mg	1200 mg	3–6 days	5–7 hours
Pregabalin ⚠ **U**			
25 mg	300 mg	3–6 days	10 hours
Clonazepam ⚠ **U**			
0.25 mg	4 mg	First dose	18–50 hours
Zopiclone ⚠ **U**			
7.5 mg	15 mg	First dose	6 hours
Zolpidem ⚠ **U**			
5 mg	10 mg	First dose	2.5 hours
Codeine phosphate U			
30 mg	90 mg	First dose	3–4 hours
Tramadol ⚠ **U**			
50 mg	200 mg	First dose	5–9 hours
Targinact® (oxycodone/naloxone) ⚠			
5 mg/2.5 mg	60 mg/30 mg	First dose	Steady state throughout day if given twice daily. Prolonged release formulation

Symbol	Meaning
🔍	This medicinal product is subject to additional monitoring
U	Unlicensed
⚠	Controlled drug (requirements vary depending on schedule. Available at: 🔗 https://www.gov.uk/government/publications/controlled-drugs-list--2/list-of-most-commonly-encountered-drugs-currently-controlled-under-the-misuse-of-drugs-legislation)

Table 28.5 Drugs used in non-REM parasomnias

Starting dose (at night unless otherwise stated)	Maximum recommended dose	Time to therapeutic effect	Half-life
Melatonin modified-release U			
0.5 mg (3 hours before bed)	6 mg (3 hours before bed)	3 hours	3–4.5 hours
Clonazepam ⚠ U			
0.25 mg	4 mg at bed	First dose	18–50 hours
Zopiclone ⚠ U			
3.75 mg	15 mg at bed	First dose	6 hours
Imipramine U			
50 mg	300 mg at bed	3–12 days	12–54 hours
Clomipramine U			
10 mg	75 mg at bed	2–3 weeks	12–36 hours
Fluoxetine U			
20 mg in the morning	60 mg in the morning	Several weeks	4–6 days
Sertraline U			
25 mg in the morning	150 mg in the morning	4.5–8.4 hours	22–36 hours

Symbol	Meaning
🖾	This medicinal product is subject to additional monitoring
U	Unlicensed
⚠	Controlled drug (requirements vary depending on schedule. Available at: 🔗 https://www.gov.uk/government/publications/controlled-drugs-list--2/list-of-most-commonly-encountered-drugs-currently-controlled-under-the-misuse-of-drugs-legislation)

Table 28.6 Drugs used in REM sleep behaviour disorder

Starting dose	Maximum recommended dosing	Time to therapeutic effect	Half-life
Melatonin modified-release U			
0.5 mg (3 hours before bed)	16 mg (3 hours before bed)	3 hours	3–4.5 hours
Clonazepam ⚠ U			
0.25 mg at bed	4 mg at bed	First dose	18–50 hours
Diazepam ⚠ U			
2 mg at bed	10 mg at bed	30–90 minutes	20–200 hours
Zopiclone ⚠ U 🖾			
3.75 mg at bed	15 mg at bed	First dose	6 hours
Pramipexole U			
0.088 mg	0.54 mg	4–10 days	8–12 hours
Rotigotine patch U			
1 mg	3 mg	1 week	5–7 hours

Symbol	Meaning
🖾	This medicinal product is subject to additional monitoring
U	Unlicensed
⚠	Controlled drug (requirements vary depending on schedule. Available at: 🔗 https://www.gov.uk/government/publications/controlled-drugs-list--2/list-of-most-commonly-encountered-drugs-currently-controlled-under-the-misuse-of-drugs-legislation)

Further reading

American Society of Health-System Pharmacists Drug Information. Available at: ⚠ https://about.medicinescomplete.com/publication/ahfs-drug-information/

Aronson AK. Meyler's Side Effects of Drugs: The International Encyclopedia of Adverse Drug Reactions and Interactions, 16th ed. Philadelphia, PA: Elsevier Science; 2015.

Buckingham R (Ed). Martindale: The Complete Drug Reference. Pharmaceutical Press; 2020. Available at: 🔗 https://about.medicinescomplete.com/publication/martindale-the-complete-drug-reference/

Sleep, the workplace, and driving

Michael Farquhar and *Adrian Williams*

Introduction

In the UK, around 3 million people, one in eight of the workforce, regularly work at night. In London, 1.6 million people—a third of the capital's workforce—regularly work evenings or nights.

They work in jobs which provide essential and emergency services, but also those which make our daytime lives more convenient. They are nurses, doctors, police, firefighters, paramedics, factory workers, transport and maintenance crews, cleaners, bakers, security guards, and call-centre workers, all ensuring our lives run like clockwork in the daytime.

There is a drive to further monetize the economy of cities like London, aiming for high-output functioning 24 hours a day, 7 days a week, to create cities which truly 'never sleep'. The economic benefits of this are estimated to be as much as £66 billion/year in the UK—however, there is a human cost to these efforts.

In 2017, the Nobel Prize in Physiology or Medicine was awarded to Hall, Rosbash, and Young for 'discoveries of molecular mechanisms controlling the circadian rhythm'. Their work illuminates the genetic and molecular workings of our body clocks, which regulate how our physiology responds to different needs and demands at different times of the day and night. Increasingly we realize how closely every aspect of our physical and mental health is tied to our circadian rhythm. When our lives are not in synchrony with our body clocks, there are significant consequences—something many of us are most familiar with when we travel around the world and become jet-lagged.

Being out of sync with our body clocks, as when jet-lagged, makes us feel disorientated, sluggish, irritable, or anxious, feeling awake and sleepy at the wrong times. We experience physical symptoms like nausea, aches, and pains. It can take days for our internal clocks to retune to the world around us and, until they do, we struggle to function.

When we ask people to work at night, physiologically we are asking them to do the same thing—to function at night as if it is day. For them, the experience of trying to function against their body clocks, of feeling jet-lagged, isn't an occasional annoyance due to travel—it's a regular fact of life.

Long-term consequences of shift work

For optimal health, it is recommended that we obtain 7–8 hours of sleep/ night, but one-third of the working population have less, a large proportion due to requirements to do shift work (regular employment outside normal daytime). Night shift workers, because of the inherent difficulty of sleeping in the day, are particularly prone to short sleep duration. In addition, there is an increasing body of evidence that suggests that the negative consequences of shift work are not purely due to sleep restriction, but are also related to circadian rhythm disruption, with resultant physiological changes, with important effects on:

- Health
- Productivity
- Safety.

Health

Lack of sufficient quality sleep (just insufficient and/or at the wrong time) is a health imperative impacting in particular on:

The cardiovascular system

According to recent meta-analyses, 7–8 hours of sleep seems to be associated with the lowest risk of cardiovascular disease. Less sleep is associated with excessive sympathetic tone and, as a consequence, diabetes mellitus, hypertension, coronary heart disease, and stroke. These are all associated with short sleep, including insomnia, and with interrupted sleep associated with SDB.

Metabolism

The epidemic of obesity has been paralleled by a significant reduction in sleep duration, with average nocturnal sleep periods having decreased from 9 hours at the beginning of the twentieth century to <8 hours now. A biologically plausible explanation has been identified through sleep deprivation experiments in which appetite increases and food choice changes related to altered leptin/ghrelin levels (leptin, a satiety hormone, being reduced and ghrelin, which stimulates appetite, being increased).

Impaired glucose tolerance has also been shown to increase with experimental short sleep duration, and, consistent with this, is found in North Sea oil rig workers at the end of their 7–10 days of night shifts.

Cancer

Short sleep duration has been associated with breast, colorectal, and prostate cancer. Epidemiological studies such as the long running Nurses' Health Study report an increased risk of these in night shift workers with a relative risk for breast cancer of 1.8 in those exposed to >20 years of rotating night shifts and a relative risk for colorectal cancer of 1.35 in those exposed to >3 nights/month for >15 years. Investigators have suggested that depressed melatonin levels may promote this association.

Productivity

Insufficient sleep is the ultimate 'performance killer'. The productivity cost of poor sleep is real, with estimates in the US in 2016 of $411 billion along with 1 million lost work days. These relate to:

- Oversleeping and arriving late at work
- Skipping work due to illness
- Fatigue-related errors, which can be especially serious in certain industries such as healthcare and transportation.

Safety

Poor sleep slows both physical and cognitive reaction times and accuracy, increasing risk for injury in the workplace.

Risk factors for occupational 'fatigue' include:

- Long work hours
- Heavy workload
- Lack of sleep
- Other medical conditions.

Tired workers become slower, less productive, and more error-prone which puts them at greater risk of a safety-related incident. This is particularly the case for those who drive as part of their job, or who commute to and from work, the problem of drowsy driving (➜ Sleepiness and driving, p. 314).

Mitigation strategies

Strategies to reduce the risks associated with shift-working broadly split into two categories: *things individuals can do* to improve their ability to cope with working around the clock, and *ways that employers can support their employees*.

Particularly for those working in emergency or critical services, professionals have a personal responsibility to ensure they are able to function as effectively as possible. However, it is absolutely essential that employers acknowledge that ensuring their staff get appropriate, adequate rest overnight, and have access to suitable facilities, is not an area where compromise can be made. The risk of fatigue-related error rapidly escalates when staff are pushed beyond their limits, especially in high-pressure environments such as hospitals.

Individual strategies

For those working night shifts as part of a rotating shift patterns, an emphasis on strengthening core sleep routine and habits is key to improving ability to work better at night (see ➔ Chapter 2 for principles of good sleep hygiene). Those who are already chronically deprived of good sleep will become vulnerable to fatigue and secondary consequences quicker.

For those working permanent night shifts, which carries with it a further increased risk of long-term health consequences, it is essential that bedroom environments in particular are optimized as much as possible for sleep.

For both groups, this means a focus on bedroom factors such as:

- Ensuring a comfortable bed
- Maximizing darkness (blackout blinds/curtains or eye masks)
- Reducing disruption from noise (ear plugs, white noise, or increasingly sophisticated noise-cancelling headphones)
- Regulating temperature as much as possible.

Night workers should also make clear that they are asleep during the daytime and those sharing daytime space with them should respect their need for sleep.

Preparing for nightshifts

Ensuring good-quality core sleep prior to starting nightshifts is probably the single most important factor in preparation. If possible, aiming to 'bank' extra sleep in the 24 hours before starting a nightshift, by having a long lie-in or by harnessing the post-lunch circadian lull to have an afternoon nap, should be attempted if possible.

During the nightshift

A consistent routine should be aimed for, with planned breaks occurring at regular times. The number of breaks permitted will vary depending on the job being worked; however, as a minimum, two 30-minute breaks for shifts lasting >9 hours should be aimed for. Planned breaks should only be omitted in exceptional circumstances.

It must be emphasized that breaks are essential for employees to be able to work safely, effectively, and efficiently and should not be viewed as an optional luxury.

For many people, short 'power-nap' periods of sleep of 15–20 minutes during night-shift breaks can have positive benefits, and help to offset some of the consequences of fatigue and circadian 'night-shift jet-lag'. A short nap will normally not result in the deeper stages of sleep, from which it is more difficult to be awoken and return to expected levels of function, being reached—this is particularly important for those working in critical emergency services. Some experimentation to find the right length of nap may be required, and it is usually helpful to set an alarm, or ask a colleague to wake you, after a set period of time. Longer periods of sleep should also be avoided as they may then further adversely affect ability to sleep the next day, which can become particularly relevant if working consecutive night shifts. If unable to power-nap, short periods of rest in a dark, quiet room may also be beneficial. Power naps of this sort are specifically endorsed in hospitals by the Royal College of Physicians, the Royal College of Nursing, and the British Medical Association.

During night-shift work, the working environment should be as bright as possible; this needs to be balanced in environments like hospitals where sleeping patients' need for night-time darkness takes priority.

Caffeine can be used to temporarily block the effects of fatigue and in-crease alertness; however, its effects tend to diminish with time and too much caffeine can lead to irritability and reduced effectiveness. Caffeine, with a half-life of 6 hours, can also reduce subsequent sleep quality and dur-ation, leading to increased fatigue on the next shift. Caffeine should there-fore be used in moderation, and preferably in the first half of the night shift. As caffeine takes around 15 minutes to take effect, often the best time to take the last caffeine shot of the shift is just before a 15–20-minute power nap—on waking, there is a double benefit from both sleep and the caffeine.

Eating at night needs to be carefully considered. Sleep deprivation and fatigue alters the pattern of secretion of the hormones leptin and ghrelin which regulate appetite and satiety, leading to increased hunger, with craving for 'comfort' foods being a frequent night-shift phenomenon—the midnight munchies! As glucose tolerance is naturally impaired at night—the body is expecting to be asleep, not eating—this contributes significantly to the car-diovascular and metabolic consequences of working at night. Increasingly, the best advice is to aim to avoid eating at all between midnight and 6 am, and when food is eaten, for this to be healthier satisfying options (e.g. soups/wholegrain sandwiches/yoghurts/fruit/salads/nuts, etc.) It is also important to ensure good hydration at night and to drink water regularly.

Finally, everyone should be aware of the 3–4 am 'dip', when the body clock is at its natural low point. Around this time, everyone's ability to func-tion is at its lowest physiological ebb. Particularly in safety-critical work, attention must be made to double and cross-check work being done at this time.

After the night shift

The major risk of immediate harm is from fatigue-induced road traffic acci-dents. If too tired to drive, shift workers should not—once awake for the functional equivalent of 16–18 hours, reaction times are likely to be similar as if at the legal drink-drive blood alcohol limit. In addition, the individual ability to assess their own degree of impairment and accurately consider risk is also impaired—a feeling often reinforced by the fact that the natural rhythm of the body lock, now moving into 'day' mode, gives the fatigued shift worker the feeling of a false 'second wind'.

Where possible public transport, or similar alternatives, should be used to get home. Shift workers should also be aware of the law around driving when tired, which assumes that any accident caused by a fatigued driver is the responsibility of the driver. Fatigued night-shift workers have been convicted of manslaughter for accidental crashes resulting in deaths when driving home after a night shift.

Wearing sunglasses on the way home can help to reduce the influence of bright light on the brain's natural circadian regulation; this should be considered with added caution if driving however.

Use of electronic screen devices should be avoided on the way home. Use of alcohol, nicotine, and caffeine should also be avoided.

The aim should be to get home and initiate sleep as soon as possible after the end of the night shift. The longer sleep onset is delayed, the less good quality sleep is likely to be achieved.

Heavy meals prior to sleep onset should be avoided but a light meal 30 minutes before going to sleep will reduce the likelihood of hunger affecting sleep quality.

On waking, aim to be exposed to bright light for at least the first 20 minutes of being awake.

Recovery

Rotating shift workers are often expected back on day shift relatively quickly after finishing nights (in hospital settings, this can be in <48 hours). It is therefore important to re-establish normal wake/sleep patterns as quickly as possible. As with all aspects of sleep, there can be a significant degree of individual variation as to best strategies.

After the final night shift, aim for a short (~90 minute—one sleep cycle) nap, with the intention being to be awake again before midday. Normal daytime activities, including exercise, preferably with exposure to natural daylight, should then be undertaken, followed by going to bed as close to the normal bedtime as possible.

On the following morning, wake time should be as close to the normal wake time as possible, with the intention again being to aim for sleep onset as close as to the normal bedtime that night as possible. A minimum of two nights of 'normal' sleep is likely to be needed to successfully re-establish the normal sleep pattern.

Judgement is likely to be impaired after a run of night shifts ... beware the post-night's spending spree!

Other considerations

Although there may be a role for use of medication (e.g. melatonin) to support staff who work at night, this should only be done following proper assessment by a medical practitioner. Self-prescribing, both of over-the-counter or internet-obtained medication or non-medication sedatives such as alcohol, should be discouraged.

Working irregular shifts, particularly night shifts, increases the risk of developing other sleep diseases and disorders as a consequence.

A small percentage of the population will have circadian clocks which are genetically incompatible with working night shifts, and may be diagnosable with shift work disorder. This is a diagnosis which should only be made by a sleep or occupational health physician following a thorough evaluation.

Employers' responsibilities

Employers must acknowledge the short- and long-term consequences of asking people to work at night, that to do so is biologically unnatural, and to put in place strategies to mitigate these risks as much as possible.

Rota design

Where rotating shift patterns are used, these should forward-rotate (morning → evening → night), reflecting the natural tendency of the intrinsic circadian clock to do the same. Numbers of transitions between day and night shifts should be minimized. Where possible, night shifts should be designed to be 8 hours or less. Adequate recovery time must be allowed after completion of a period of night-shift working.

Education

Basic education about the importance of good sleep, strategies to improve core sleep routine and habits, as well as specific teaching about how to cope better with working at nights should routinely be offered to all staff asked to work at night.

Rest/breaks

Rest and break entitlements should be clear, and employers should ensure a positive attitude towards these, with an emphasis that breaks are not a luxury and are essential both to optimize job-related performance, but also to reduce short- and long-term health consequences to staff.

Facilities

Staff should have access to appropriate rest/break facilities during night shifts, including access to hot and healthy food options, and to spaces which support 'power-naps' during breaks.

Safe driving

Where employees drive home after a night shift, there should be conscious consideration by those on the day shift as to whether they are safe to do so. If they are felt to be unsafe, provision should either be made for them to sleep on-site until they are safe to drive, or for alternative arrangements to be made for them to get home (this is now a legal requirement of National Health Service employers for junior doctors).

Screening

All staff who regularly work night shifts should be offered annual occupational health screening for primary sleep disorders.

Sleepiness and driving

Alertness is critical for safe driving, which is a complex task involving distinct cognitive, motor, and decision-making skills. Because sleepiness can affect some or all of these, it is not surprising that excessive sleepiness, and not necessarily falling asleep, would be associated with an increase in motor vehicle accidents. One in five fatal crashes involve a drowsy driver, and one in two fatal crashes involve commercial heavy goods vehicle drivers.

Epidemiology of sleep-related vehicle accidents

The National Sleep Foundation, and others, have reported:
- 60% of drivers admitting to driving while feeling sleepy at some time
- 40% to have nodded off at some time
- 25% to have nodded off once a month
- 15% to have nodded off once a week
- Self-reported sleepiness is associated with a 2.5 times increased risk of accidents.

Effect of drowsiness on driving

Drowsiness/sleepiness impairs cognitive function, including:
- Judgement
- Attention
- Executive function
- Reaction time
- Coordination.

The impact on cognitive function is compounded by microsleeps, temporary lapses in consciousness/awareness during which the EEG shows theta activity superimposed on background alpha activity or wakefulness. People are unaware, but there may be head nodding, slow eyelid closure, and eyelid drooping.

Relationship to time slept

After 17–18 hours of continuous wake, results of psychomotor vigilance testing (a test of sustained attention and vigilance) resemble that seen in drivers with a blood alcohol content of 0.05%, the legal limit for driving in many European countries (Fig. 29.1).

Relation to circadian factors

Sleep propensity is greatest at 3–5 am and also 2–4 pm, driven by robust circadian mechanisms and reflected in the increased number of sleep-related accidents at those times.

Who is at risk?

- Teenagers
- Patients with sleep disorders, including OSA. Having sleep apnoea increases the risk of driving accidents two- to threefold. Factors associated are age, an increase of BMI, a high AHI, and severity of hypoxaemia. Sleepiness is predictive in some, but not all, indicating that absence of sleepiness does not eliminate risk
- Other disorders are not exempt, although data are limited. Those with insomnia are affected, for example

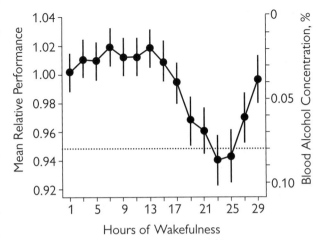

Fig. 29.1 A plot of mean relative performance and blood alcohol concentration equivalent against hours of wakefulness showing that the effects of moderate sleep loss on performance are clearly similar to moderate alcohol intoxication.

Reproduced with permission from Dawson, Drew, and Reid, Kathryn, Fatigue, alcohol and performance impairment, (17 July 1997) Nature; 388: 235.

- Commercial drivers. Sleep-deprived driving is a major problem in commercial transportation and in the military—20% of commercial pilots and 18% of train operators have admitted to making a serious error due to fatigue. Commercial truck drivers are especially susceptible to drowsy driving. A recent study of 80 long-haul truck drivers in the US and Canada found that drivers averaged <5 hours of sleep per day. The National Transportation Safety Board reported that drowsy driving was likely the cause of more than half of crashes leading to a truck driver's death. For each truck driver fatality, another three to four people are killed.

Evaluation of drowsy drivers

- Identify and treat underlying causes
- Identify high-risk behaviours such as lack of sleep, use of sedatives, or occupation
- Many countries have medical standards that include specific questions about sleep apnoea and other sleep disorders, but there are no unified legal regulations. In the US, the National Sleep Foundation recommends objective testing for those with those with a BMI >35 kg/m². Subjective assessments seem to be insufficient; e.g. in an Australian study of 514 truckers, assessed at two truck stops, 12% admitted to sleepiness and 4.4% to a diagnosis of sleep apnoea, but on testing, 45% had sleep apnoea.

Prevention and countermeasures

- Recognition of drowsy driving:
  - Difficulty focusing
  - Frequent blinking
  - Heavy eyelids
  - Daydreaming
  - Difficulty remembering the last few miles or a missed exit
  - Yawning
  - Head bobbing
  - Drifting lanes
- Planning ahead:
  - Adequate prior sleep
  - Avoid time of day when sleepiness is more likely to be evident
  - Brief naps and caffeine intake
- Treating known OSA
- Stimulants, e.g. modafinil—a study of eight individuals after being awake all night and given modafinil 300 mg versus placebo, showed a reduction in lane deviations but not off-road deviations. This is not licensed in the UK
- Other:
  - Autotactile lane markings i.e. rumble strips, which reduce road traffic accidents by 20–50%
  - Regulation-permissible wake hours, as in New York State.

Legal aspects

In all societies and legal jurisdictions, it is accepted that permission to drive vehicles is not a right but a privilege. That privilege comes with responsibilities, one of which is to be fully alert and attentive when in control of a vehicle. Being sleepy at the wheel is therefore not acceptable, nor permitted.

The actual rules that govern such behaviour vary from country to country and state to state in the US for example, and in all cases, physicians should be aware of local rules regarding driving and notification in the context of sleep disorders. However, the 'Position Statement on Driving and Obstructive Sleep Apnoea' (2018) from the British Thoracic Society is a worthwhile example, and is reproduced in part here:

WHEN IS SLEEPINESS EXCESSIVE AND LIKELY TO ADVERSELY AFFECT DRIVING?

The Epworth Sleepiness Scale (ESS) alone is unlikely to be adequate, as it is subjective.

The American Thoracic Society Practice Guidelines offer useful guidance. They emphasise the importance of the clinician identifying a high-risk driver by direct questioning. They suggest a high-risk driver is one who has moderate to severe daytime sleepiness (suggesting an ESS of >17/24) plus a recent motor vehicle collision (MVC) or a near-miss attributable to sleepiness, fatigue or inattention. They found no compelling evidence to restrict driving privileges in patients with OSA if there had not been a motor vehicle crash or equivalent event.

People who experience head nodding, hitting the rumble strip, regularly using alerting manoeuvres such as keeping the windows open, stopping for a drink or to stretch, or listening to loud music are more likely to have impaired driving due to sleepiness.

Some specialists impose restrictions on driving, suggesting 'some people find they can avoid excessive sleepiness by driving short distances only, driving for less than an hour, driving at times of day when they recognise they are most alert and ensuring adequate night-time sleep plus daytime naps'.

Specialist tests of alertness and driving simulation may help to inform these discussions, but do not have any legal standing, and there is no evidence that they predict the likelihood of MVCs.

Historically, the MSLT and the MWT have been the primary objective tests used for the measurement of sleepiness and alertness, respectively. The MWT procedure requires the subject, with EEG recorded, to sit up in a chair in a quiet and dimly lit room with instructions to stay awake. Vocalizations and movements are not allowed. Four or five trials are given, beginning 1.5 to 3 hours after awakening and recurring every 2 hours thereafter. Each trial is terminated after 40 minutes if no sleep has occurred, or immediately after sleep onset. It is reasoned that instructing patients to stay awake rather than to allow themselves to fall asleep is a more accurate reflection of their ability to function and maintain alertness in common situations of inactivity, such as driving. However, studies of normal individuals are few and small, and an abnormal MSL is currently difficult to define.

In general, a diagnosis of excessive sleepiness should be made with extreme care and with as much clinical information as possible. Based on current evidence, the MSL should not be the sole criterion for determining sleepiness or for certifying a diagnosis or response to treatment. Interpretation of test results should be made within the context of the individual patient history and as part of other medical information and testing.

Conclusion

Both sleep deprivation and circadian rhythm disruption have serious repercussions. However, these are not limited to the individual but have a wider relevance to society at large, with regard to health, productivity, and public safety. This is particularly pertinent to those in safety-critical roles and drivers. Individuals, organizations, and society all have a duty to ensure adequate quality and quantity of sleep to mitigate these risks.

Further reading

British Thoracic Society Position Statement: Driving and Obstructive Sleep Apnoea. 2018. Available at: ℘ https://www.brit-thoracic.org.uk/document-library/governance-and-policy-documents/position-statements/position-statement-on-driving-and-obstructive-sleep-apnoea/

Driving and Vehicle Licensing Agency (UK). Assessing Fitness to Drive – A Guide for Medical Professionals. 2021. Available at: ℘ http://www.gov.uk/government/publications/assessing-fitness-to-drive-a-guide-for-medical-professionals

Horrocks N, Pounder R. Working the night shift: preparation, survival and recovery—a guide for junior doctors. RCP Working Group. Clin Med (Lond) 2006;6(1):61–7.

Kecklund G, Azelsson J. Health consequences of shift work and insufficient sleep. BMJ. 2016;355:i5210.

Lee M, Howard M, Horrey W, et al. High risk of near-crash driving events following night-shift work. Proc Natl Acad Sci U S A. 2016;113(1):176–81.

Index